D1275788

Relief
Is in the
Stretch

Relief
Is in the
Stretch

END BACK PAIN
THROUGH YOGA

Loren Fishman, MD
Carol Ardman

W. W. Norton & Company
New York • London

For information about permission to reproduce selections from this book,
write to Permissions, W. W. Norton & Company, Inc., 500 Fifth Avenue, New York, NY 10110

Manufacturing by The Maple-Vail Book Manufacturing Group
Book design by Molly Heron
Production manager: Amanda Morrison

Library of Congress Cataloging-in-Publication Data

Fishman, Loren.
Relief is in the stretch : end back pain through yoga /
Loren Fishman, Carol Ardman.— 1st ed.
p. cm.
Summary: "Offers specific yoga techniques to cure or control back pain and sciatica
according to its cause"—Provided by publisher.
Includes bibliographical references and index.
ISBN 0-393-05833-6 (hardcover)
1. Back pain—Exercise therapy. 2. Hatha yoga—Therapeutic use. I. Ardman, Carol. II. Title.
RD771.B217F5683 2005
617.5'64062—dc22
2004025223

W. W. Norton & Company, Inc.
500 Fifth Avenue, New York, N.Y. 10110
www.wwnorton.com

W. W. Norton & Company Ltd.
Castle House, 75/76 Wells Street, London W1T 3QT

1 2 3 4 5 6 7 8 9 0

TO MY BELOVED TEACHER, B.K.S. IYENGAR

In 1973 I was a young man wandering in India, seeking answers. I had heard of Mr. Iyengar and had done every pose in his book as well as I could, twice daily, for about a year. I was also contemplating becoming a doctor.

I arrived in Pune at siesta time. I went to Mr. Iyengar's house and knocked on his door. To my surprise, he opened it.

"What do you want?" he demanded rather grumpily.

"I want to learn your yoga."

"Why?"

"Because I want to heal," I blurted out.

"That's my great thing!" he said. "Come in."

My debt to Mr. Iyengar extends beyond words. However, it must be stated that I (and not he) am responsible for everything in the text.

CONTENTS

NOTE TO READERS

This book is not a substitute for medical advice and assistance. The judgment of individual therapists and physicians who know you is essential. It is in this setting of personal, expert attention that yoga was developed, and the setting for which it has always been intended.

ACKNOWLEDGMENTS

We would like to thank the many friends and professionals who contributed medical, yoga, and editorial advice to this book. Tova Ovadia, PT; Carole Lewis, PT, PhD; Caroline Konnoth, PT; Barry Pinchoff, MD; James Dillard, MD; and Donald Cohen, MD, have stimulated our thought and made invaluable suggestions.

Christine Saudek, MS, PT, and certified senior Iyengar yoga teacher, shared her expertise, reading our manuscript for accuracy during the final stages of writing and revision, asking difficult questions and attending to every detail.

Experts in yoga and alternative medicine have been generous with their time and ideas. Special thanks are due to Sally Hess, model par excellence, for her patience and tireless technical and editorial work. We are also grateful to Mary Dunn, Ellen Saltenstall, Joan White, Victor Oppenheimer, Leslie Kaminoff (the Breathing Project, New York City), Pamela Miles (Institute for the Advancement of Complementary Therapies), Eric Small, Sheldon Lewis, Paul Frediani (Sports Athletics), Ellen Peterman, Jon Keller, and Vidya Albrink.

For editorial help and general support without which this book would not have been possible, we would like to express our gratitude to Amy Hertz, Ellen Levine, Jill Bialosky, Jane Bernstein, Warren Sidall, Tom Murtha, Mark Rudman, Eileen Stukane, Sheila Weller, and John Cooney.

PART I

Yoga and Back Pain

CHAPTER 1

What Is Yoga and Why Yoga for Back Pain?

Many people experience back pain from time to time. Whether this pain is severe and chronic or mild and short-lived, it often causes misery and curtails everyday activities.[1] Why practice yoga for back pain? Yoga has been associated with healing through the millennia. It is without cost, self-administered, and silent, and it demands no equipment beyond a pillow, a belt, or a chair. Yoga relieves pain and promotes calm to endure any pain that remains. It can address back pain generally, through prevention, and directly with attention to the specific cause of existing pain. No special beliefs are required in the practice of yoga.

What Is Yoga?

Yoga means "yoke" (a link, a harness that joins together) or "unity." This unity refers to the oneness of body and mind. The purpose of yoga is to bring together the body and mind to create harmony, or well-being. The word *yoga* also means "discipline" or "effort."

Some people think of yoga as an art; others call it a science. Most would agree that although it is associated with Hinduism, it is a secular practice that can be done by individuals of any faith or no faith. I like to think of yoga as a system of behavior that encompasses mankind's social context; that is, it exists in a social environment, influencing and being influenced by the community around it. Certainly yoga has gathered devoted practitioners from many different faiths and lands.

The classical form of yoga has eight limbs, or branches, the first two of which are relevant for anyone who considers using yoga to aid in the healing process, to relieve back pain or any other type of pain.

Universal moral commandments having to do with our relations with others, called *Yama,* constitute the first limb. These are concerned with nonviolence, truthfulness, not stealing, temperance, and noncovetousness. The second limb of yoga, *Niyama,* contains individual moral directives, including purity, contentment, austerity, introspection, and dedication to a higher being.

There is no question in my mind that *Yama* and *Niyama* serve the purpose of anyone seeking healing. Following these codes—living an uncomplicated life, with dignity, purpose, and compassion—is very strong medicine. As the gyroscope's internal motion resists deflecting influence, reasonably disciplined striving toward personal improvement creates its own momentum.

Asanas, or "postures," make up the third limb of yoga. In the West, these positions—lotus position, headstand, and so on—are typically identified with yoga. Hatha (physical) yoga is made up of asanas. When I was in India, Mr. Iyengar demonstrated various asanas for his classes; these poses had been practiced and refined for thousands of years. Within the various schools of yoga, the style of these asanas differs; also, some poses are still evolving. Some asanas have biological names based on the gestalt of the position. The Tree and the Scorpion are examples of these. Others are named for their "attitude," for example, after gods in Hindu mythology: Hanumanasana or Virabhadrasana. A third group of asanas is known for the anatomical parts that figure most prominently in their execution, such as the headstand or arm balance.

The fourth limb is *Pranayama,* which concerns the apparatus and technique of breathing. This practice is used in a number of respiratory and psychiatric conditions but also to help the student progress beyond mere physical health and toward a state of liberation. Many yogis believe that breathing is the bridge between the body and the soul.

Pratyahara, control of the senses (desires), is the fifth limb. *Dharana,* the sixth limb, focuses an individual's mind and promotes concentration. Next, *Dhyana* is a blissful state in which one selflessly devotes one's time and energy to seeing the spiritual essences and giving all of one's resources for the betterment of the world. Finally, *Samadhi* is the attainment of liberation or enlightenment.

In the type of yoga you will likely be practicing, "the yogi frees himself from physical disabilities and mental distractions by practicing asanas," as Mr. Iyengar wrote in his classic book, *Light on Yoga.* It isn't an accident that one of the first textbooks on yoga was written by Patanjali, who lived thousands of years ago and is believed to have been a physician.

Although all of the hundreds of different yoga postures are aimed at improving health and increasing personal calm, some poses are noted to have specific effects and are considered to be especially appropriate for individual conditions such as back pain.

Why Practice Yoga for Back Pain?

My friend Tom provides a dramatic example of the way yoga can speed the healing process. Tom was an eighteen-year-old learning to rock climb when he had an accident that involved a long fall from the top of a cliff. He was lucky to survive; unluckily, he cracked two of his lower vertebrae. Tom's physician happened to be a native of India, and a yoga practitioner. He knew that the boy's injuries could be treated through yoga. At first he taught Tom how to sit properly, so that his spine was properly aligned. This, Tom remembers, was instrumental not only in alleviating his pain but also in facilitating his eventual cure.

Prevention

At one time or another almost everyone suffers from back pain, the cause of more lost days of work than anything but the common cold, so the world has turned to secondary prevention as a principal means of addressing it.[2] Yoga is an ideal preventive for those who have either chronic or occasional pain. Tom is an example of someone who learned that yoga can heal, but even now he has to take care of his back and his whole person to prevent old injuries from flaring up. He accomplishes that with yoga.

Secondary prevention involves taking steps to avoid the consequences of a condition. For example, currently there is no cure for diabetes mellitus. But if diabetics carefully regulate their serum glucose and diet, then neuropathy, cardiovascular complications, peripheral vascular disease, and ocular problems can be minimized or avoided.[3] This applies in full force to lower back pain, where reduced activity leads to stiff muscles and joints and to weakness, which are the main causes of *chronic* back pain.

Overall prevention is impossible. For example, you can't prevent all colds and flu; you can't prevent the accident that causes a broken leg; you can't keep all misfortunes from happening. What you can do, however, is reduce their frequency, severity, and duration. For colds and flu, for example, washing your hands and strengthening your immune system with a healthy diet and lifestyle may make a difference in how often you contract a cold or flu, how badly you suffer, and how long the illness lasts.

Paradoxically, for back pain, prevention constitutes cure. In practicing prevention, your goal is to stop pain from becoming chronic. Yoga does this in eight ways: stretching muscles to reduce spasm and increase flexibility, strengthening muscles and bones, increasing range of motion, sharpening focus, heightening self-awareness, and producing calm. It also improves balance and agility.

You can practice yoga just about anywhere, without spending money, without props, without making noise, and without wearing special garb or giving up your beliefs.

Reducing Spasm

There are two types of sense organs that record the tension within: One type inside the muscle fibers themselves is called intrafusal fibers. These actually have their own tiny muscles that adjust the tension according to the larger muscle's length. Intrafusal fibers are embedded within the muscles themselves, and when tension increases, either through external pull or because other muscles are contracting, they influence muscles to contract. When there is stress on them, the muscles react by tensing. The intrafusal fibers are dynamic. Tiny muscle fibers inside each intrafusal unit adjust the sensing mechanism to the current conditions of the muscle. Therefore they have a large immediate effect when you move, but that effect gets weaker and weaker as they adjust and as a result movement or tension continues.

The golgi tendon organs, on the other hand, give off a constant inhibitory signal that varies only according to the tension on the muscle. The golgi tendon organs (located in the tendons) cause the muscles to relax when they are stretched. They are static. They produce a constant, unchanging level of signals to the central nervous system to relax the muscle.

At first, the intrafusal fibers actually intensify resistance to stretch, increasing the amount of spasm that is present. But over a short time, their own adjustment mechanism cuts down their input. Usually in less than two minutes the force of the intrafusal fibers falls below the relaxing influence of the golgi tendon organs. Cumulatively, the forces that cause muscles to contract—to get tight when stretched—decrease. The constant inhibitory influence of the golgi tendon organs prevails. The result of this is that stretching a muscle and keeping it in that extended position for any length of time allows relaxation to overtake excitability. The muscle relaxes. Then there is a domino effect that may travel elsewhere in the body, making other muscles become less tense. When you begin a yoga pose, the relaxation that results when the golgi tendon organs go into action is masked at first by the effect of the excitable intrafusal fibers, but that effect falls off quite quickly, while the damping action of the golgi tendon organs continues as long as you are in the pose.[4] Slow and steady wins the day. It is one essential way you can help your body to counter spasm and reduce back pain.

This strategy of staying in a given stretch position for a length of time relies on a reflex, a natural and "hardwired" mechanism that functions at the spinal cord level. It works without our consent. Although we set out to do it on purpose, the effect is mediated on a wholly unconscious level. There is no question that the calm it brings has effects farther up in the central nervous system. We will encounter that benefit of yoga soon enough. But we should first consider another reflex mechanism that can be used to relax involuntarily constricted muscles in spasm.

Every time you flex your elbow, you use your biceps. And every time the biceps contracts and flexes the elbow, its opposite, the triceps, which straightens the elbow when it contracts, must relax and stretch to allow the elbow to bend. Two muscles in this relationship are called "agonist" and "antagonist," depending upon which is doing the contracting. There are many such pairs in the body, of course, and the absence of either partner of the set, through amputation or paralysis, for example, often brings severe spasm to the one that remains.

This opposition is obviously extremely useful. What good is a hand that can grasp if the fingers cannot be opened? These pairs of muscles, mutually dependent for their utility, require precise coordination. Another reflex simplifies the operation: Contraction of one member of the pair works unconsciously to relax the other member of the pair. So as you raise your head by contracting the muscles of the back of the neck, relaxation takes place in the muscles beside the throat that would bring your head down.

Yoga uses this simple but powerful mechanism in many ways. For example, bending forward by contracting the stomach muscles simultaneously relaxes the antagonistic muscles of the lumbar spine. Holding that forward position for a length of time, keeping the abdominal muscles contracted, invokes the relaxing effect of stretching both the golgi tendon organs and the agonist-antagonist mechanism, formidable adversaries of the painful back spasm that we want to vanquish.

Flexibility

A joint in the human body is really miraculous, moving back and forth, as many as hundreds of thousands of times a day for as long as a hundred years, without ever getting stuck! When something does go wrong, however, wear and tear may take place and range of motion may become limited.

Through well-known stretching postures, yoga extends the range of motion of the joints. The inside of the joint capsule, which surrounds the joint much the way a gasket surrounds the juncture between the sink and the faucet, secretes a thick, lubricating substance called synovial fluid, which greases the joint, lubricates it, and allows it to move freely and smoothly. If tendons, ligaments, or muscles associated with the joint become tight, there may not be enough fluid to keep it working properly. Movement may be limited, or there may be pain. No studies have been done on the effect of yoga on synovial fluid, but yoga can safely enlarge the capsule and therefore allow it to continue to function as a secreter and container of synovial fluid.[5]

Ligaments around the joint are made of basically the same material as the capsule, but they are much stronger. Their function is to protect the capsule against overly vigorous movement or movement beyond the normal range of motion. Hatha yoga can stretch ligaments little by little if they become tight or stiff.

Apart from resolving spasm, yoga can also stretch otherwise tense or shortened muscles, changing their length through the continuous pressure exerted on them when an individual attains and holds a particular pose. The stretch itself may engender some discomfort. While that isn't always entirely pleasant, the pain does serve a purpose. It calls attention to the problem area and is likely to provide motivation for an individual to gain control of, say, a particular muscle. Through repeated effort one learns to make that muscle relax. A relaxed muscle can stretch farther. That is key. After controlling the muscle spasm that is so common in back pain, yoga then stretches the muscle farther, so that more movement is possible with less pain. Around joints, yoga increases range of motion; joints at one remove from the painful one adapt by increasing their range of motion to take on some of the strain from the places that are actually producing the pain, allowing them to heal.

Strength

There are two ways yoga increases strength. First, as with any exercise, muscles get stronger when holding a specific position for any length of time, even for a few seconds, because the body has to fight against the forces of gravity to keep itself in position. In this way, yoga is a little like lifting weights.[6] The counterforce is the weight of your own body and the resistance to movement that different muscles and joints provide. But yoga often increases strength isometrically. Isometric exercise takes place when muscles contract without joints moving. For example, if you lace your fingers together and then try to pull your hands apart, your muscles will contract without any movement taking place. Isometric exercise increases strength with stunning efficiency.[7]

Unlike some activities, the goal of yoga is to gain control, not lose it. Students of yoga who do poses, or asanas, develop personal techniques for relaxing their muscles. These techniques are enhanced by involuntary processes. Nerves have what is called a refractory period. After conducting signals, there is a short period during which they cannot be stimulated to carry any signal, no matter how strong the stimulus. And muscle fibers fatigue from contraction. If one stimulates a previously resting nerve fiber, attached to a calm muscle fiber, it is likely to arouse a maximally powerful contraction. If fifty workmen have the job of moving a heavy block, and some are pulling while others rest from having pulled a moment ago, they will not be as effective as fifty workmen who all pull at once and together. Not only is the muscle stronger; its fibers contract more simultaneously: Strength is more effectively utilized.[8]

Strength is not only a matter of muscles being strong and all their fibers contracting simultaneously; strength is also related to strong bones. The unorthodox and quite sharp pulls that tendons and ligaments make on the bones in the course of doing yoga have been shown in humans and animals to arrest and possibly to reverse osteoporosis.[9]

Calm

It's well known that stress can contribute to back pain and that yoga reduces stress. Yoga, however, approaches this in a way unfamiliar to Westerners. We believe our minds cause our bodies to move, our brains sending signals down nerve pathways to our muscles. And, of course, that's true. However, in yoga, the opposite also applies. The state induced by yoga in our bodies calms our minds.

Breathing exercises are another resource of yoga that produce calm. These exercises are actually an entire realm of yoga as large as

all of hatha, or physical, yoga. Breathing, or Pranayama, is the rhyth-
mical and sophisticated use of one's breath to produce a specific
effect. There are centers in the brain that control inhaling and exhaling. Gaining some mastery of these centers seems to control not just
breathing itself but a number of other rhythmic and alternating patterns in the brain that, when regulated, produce salutary effects.
The individual practicing Pranayama not only becomes calm
through breathing in and breathing out regularly; the calm also
seems to "spread" through the central nervous system, giving a
model of mastery that can be replicated elsewhere in the nervous
system. When this is done, it produces an overwhelming level of
calm and self-control.

Herbert Benson, MD, of Harvard Medical School described this
type of breathing, which is taught in the mantra meditation used in
transcendental meditation, in his 1975 book, *The Relaxation
Response*.[10] Basing his thesis on studies at Boston's Beth Israel Hospital and Harvard Medical School, Dr. Benson showed that relaxation
techniques such as meditation have immense physical benefits,
from lowered blood pressure to a reduction in heart disease, and he
made these techniques accessible to everyone. Other introductory
texts on Pranayama have been written by B.K.S. Iyengar and Mira
Mehta.[11]

Self-Knowledge

There are two more interlocking ways in which yoga helps, especially if you have back pain. A type of self-understanding comes
from practicing yoga. Both watching your own reactions to pain and
stress and experiencing your own determination to gain mastery
over the asanas contribute to your knowledge of yourself. You gain
simple understanding of the way your own body works and the
things that are better and worse for it, the things that are easier to do
and more difficult. This is knowledge in the usual sense of knowing
that your back bends only to a certain extent, but it is also knowledge in a deeper sense. You become more than acquainted with
yourself; you become familiar. Being familiar with your own body—
knowing what you can and cannot do—is a cardinal way to avoid
back pain in the first place.

And now for the final advantages to achieving calm. In addition to reducing the drone of anxiety in the background of one's life and increasing the understanding of yourself, yoga contains a means of keeping yourself from getting too excited. Through the practice of yoga you learn how to avoid getting yourself into desperate situations in which you are likely to injure your back or injure it further. Far from trivial, the most important thing in treating back pain (because you can't always avoid it) is to prevent it from becoming chronic. Yoga is the best means I know of for reducing back pain to manageable levels, if not completely abolishing it, and keeping it from becoming a dominant factor in your life.

There are now scientific programs to prove how and how well yoga "works."[12] Yoga actually increases your sense of well-being and self-reliance and is a strong combatant to depression, which may lead to increased somatization of any symptom. But basically it is for aesthetic reasons that people embrace yoga—because of the combination of humility, kindness, consideration, strength, temperance, generosity, and expecting much from yourself and little from others that attracts people to yoga. Essentially people do it not only because they believe they should, but because they want to.

The idea of being able to coordinate one muscle with another presupposes familiarity with one's body, strength and flexibility, focus and self-knowledge. In addition, yoga promotes balance, symmetry, and grace.

CHAPTER 2

Styles of Yoga

A few weeks ago I ran into my next-door neighbor as we were coming home from work. "I'm thinking of beginning to do yoga," she said. "My back aches sometimes. Maybe it's what everybody calls aches and pains. Also, I want to keep in shape. The problem is I have no idea how to choose which yoga to do. There are so many different types, and it's hard to remember and pronounce the names. Do you have any suggestions?"

Let me emphasize, if you have severe back pain, numbness, weakness, or trouble controlling bowel and bladder functions, you should not sign up for a yoga class but should first get a diagnosis and then, if appropriate, find a yoga therapist. However, many people who are not having an attack of acute pain or who just want to keep their backs fit, do want to take classes, and they want to do it safely.

It is a tribute to Patanjali's brilliance and the specific efficacy of yoga that it has remained so unified over thousands of years. Nevertheless, there are many different styles of yoga, partially because it has become so widespread. And the many variations on the theme are extremely confusing. If you're having a similar difficulty in choosing a place to begin your practice, here's a little guidance.

Hatha yoga is what is commonly practiced here in the West. It's often thought of as a combination of physical yoga, or asanas, and breathing exercises, or Pranayama. If you are considering doing yoga that is identified only as "hatha," it probably has elements of several yoga styles, some of which I discuss below. My advice is not to do yoga that is designated only as hatha without finding out:

- how strenuous the workout will be
- how many poses are done in what period of time
- the level of difficulty of the poses
- how and where the teacher was trained
- what kind of yoga the teacher does
- whether there is attention to physical problems like back pain
- whether meditation is included in the lesson

Now here's some history I hope will help bring the yoga picture more into focus for you. The grandfather of modern yoga, and the person who spearheaded today's main currents of practice, was an Indian man called Krishnamacharya, who died at the age of 101 in 1997. A scholar, a healer, a synthesizer of ancient wisdom, Krishamacharya was also a great teacher. Three of his students started three of the main branches of yoga that are popular in the West today. One of them, B.K.S. Iyengar, was my teacher and the first of Krishnamacharya's students to become well known. The other two were Patabi Jois, who founded a movement called Ashtanga yoga, and Desikachar, Krishnamacharya's son, who carries on the Viniyoga tradition. Many other styles of yoga spring from these three, but not all the styles of yoga I mention here are from that tradition.

Iyengar yoga is known for its focus on the accuracy of the poses. This is the school of yoga that takes precision seriously. For instance, you might spend not minutes, but hours, and finally years studying the four corners of the feet—where they are exactly, how to become aware of them, and how to use them to achieve balance and symmetry. This particular subject of the feet, by the way, is interesting theoretically, as are many other anatomical subjects studied by

Iyengar yogis, but the subject of feet is also one you may find important if you have low back pain.

Therapeutics—all kinds of healing—are essential to Mr. Iyengar's approach. There is attention to alignment, making sure that the muscle that ought to bear the weight really is bearing the weight and is being well supported. Students of Iyengar yoga are taught to sit and stand with exactitude. This attention to the precise positioning of the body, with the goal of symmetry, balance, and calm, is the prelude to meditation. Breathing as conscious movement is the bridge between the tranquil body and the meditative mind. Meditation is much more than merely being quiet.

In Iyengar yoga, you do a posture. Then you hold the posture. After that you go on to the next posture. A good Iyengar teacher will stimulate your interest by coming back again and again to specific postures that are being explored and may be improved. In this way, a series of classes can be an exciting experience intellectually as well as physically and spiritually.

While Mr. Iyengar himself and those who teach his yoga are known for being anatomically sophisticated, his techniques build strength and flexibility on a firm foundation. In addition to his first book about physical yoga, *Light on Yoga*, Mr. Iyengar has written many other books, including *Light on Pranayama: The Yogic Art of Breathing*. He is also a scholar of Hindu scripture.

Iyengar teachers are particularly well suited to working with people who have back pain. They must undergo rigorous, lengthy training, and they have a reputation for being well prepared and competent. Their credentialing process assures that those who are designated to teach this type of yoga are extremely well trained.

Patabi Jois is the father of the popular Ashtanga yoga, taught in many health clubs. This active, strenuous practice may be very athletic and therefore not appropriate for those with back pain. It consists of six series of sequential postures of increasing difficulty. Breathing—in this method called vinyasa—is essential, and while it isn't exactly classical Pranayama, students do synchronize their breathing with the poses and use it to link one pose to the next. Ashtanga yoga is meant to be fast. The idea is that the practitioner builds up internal heat that culminates in a purifying sweat. Breathing is an elemental part of Ashtanga, and the practitioner must focus on it, often putting less emphasis on precision of body placement.

Since Ashtanga doesn't focus on accuracy in the way that Iyengar practice does, it may be most appropriate for people who want a thorough, rather aerobic workout. Power yoga, also taught in many gyms and health clubs, grew out of Ashtanga. While the Ashtanga practice is based in India, Richard Freeman is a respected teacher in Boulder, Colorado. He has a video, books, and a Web site: *www.yogaworkshop.com*.

Ironically the least known of Krishnamacharya's three students who have become famous teachers themselves is his own son. Desikachar has dedicated his life to passing on his father's teachings, which reflect the way yoga was studied and practiced thousands of years ago. Viniyoga concentrates on the individual, using poses, breathing, meditation, ritual, and prayer to promote and maintain physical health and to help in the quest for self-realization. The thrust of Viniyoga is that yoga is something you do with yourself. It's personal. This is one of the main reasons Viniyoga is so well suited to therapeutics.

There are Viniyoga teachers who have instructed students for years but have always done it one-on-one and have never taught a class. If you do this type of yoga, your relationship with your teacher is personal. As you are taught, the pose is customized, individualized for you and your needs in that very moment. It has been said that Viniyoga "troubleshoots" your body. It's about the individual working toward a goal. Because Viniyoga involves working so closely, student to teacher, there are many people who haven't heard of it. If you would like to find out more, you can contact the American Viniyoga Institute in Hawaii (808-572-1414) or go to *www.viniyoga.com*.

There are several popular types of yoga that are outgrowths of the three I've just talked about. One I consider valuable, especially for anyone who has back pain, is Anusara yoga (*www.anusara.com*). John Friend, a former student of Mr. Iyengar, founded this highly respected movement in 1997. The word *Anusara* means "flowing with grace." Mr. Friend's approach focuses on outer and inner body alignment, and respects each student's abilities and limitations. Practitioners consider Anusara safe because it has the accuracy of Iyengar practice but is more lighthearted and less perfectionistic.

People who have back pain are enthusiastic about the therapeutic results of Anusara. Teachers do not try to "correct" or "fix" the mistakes of students, but instead try to "enhance and reveal the beauty and divine qualities that are already present." However, detailed corrections are offered. The practice is considered "heart oriented," and students are encouraged to express their core, or to shine out through individual postures. Anusara teacher training, like Iyengar teacher training, is lengthy, rigorous, and thorough, as is its credentialing process.

It would take a book to cover every style of yoga and describe it, but there are a few more I will mention briefly.

Bikram yoga takes place in a room with a temperature of approximately 100 degrees. This is meant to warm the muscles so they can stretch and also to replicate the environment in which yoga began. The sequence of twenty-six traditional poses is done vigorously, producing "cleansing sweat." Is this type of yoga safe for everyone? Probably not.

Kripalu is a three-stage yoga considered by some experts to be "feel good" yoga that is customized for Westerners. In the first stage, postural alignment and coordination of breath and movement are stressed. Some feel that accuracy is not a high priority, but this style of yoga does help people begin stretching in a way that is not dangerous.

Integral Yoga, developed by Swami Satchitananda, is a gentle practice enlivened by chanting. This practice includes hatha yoga, selfless service, meditation, and prayer, and influenced Dr. Dean Ornish's work in reversing heart disease and Dr. Michael Lerner's noted Commonweal Cancer Help program.[1]

Sivananda is a highly respected yoga practice that is also widespread. As in other schools of yoga, there is emphasis on mind/body work. Its hatha yoga practice consists of twelve basic postures that are intended to increase spinal strength and flexibility. Chanting, breathing, and meditation are also essential. However, it is difficult to adapt this style to individual physical problems.

Svaroopa-style yoga uses classical yoga poses to open the deeper muscles around the spine, with the goal of helping the whole body to relax and move more freely. Svaroopa-style yoga was developed by Rama Berch, founder of Master Yoga Academy in La Jolla, California. Starting at the tailbone and working up through the spine, supported poses are meant to help contracted areas of the body to release. There are five levels of training, culminating in certification as a Svaroopa Yoga Therapist and as an Advanced Svaroopa Yoga Teacher.

Phoenix Rising Yoga Therapy, headquartered in Stockbridge, Massachusetts, blends releasing tension with stretching and assisted movement in supported yoga postures with dialogue that is aimed at helping practitioners let go of old emotions and beliefs that may be manifesting as chronic aches and pains. Phoenix Rising also has thorough teacher training.

CHAPTER 3

Doing Yoga

Yoga is generally practiced every day, sometimes every other day. In chronic illness, yoga is often the opposite of medicine. A famous guru used to contrast medications and yoga, saying that at first medicines are like heaven, but after a while they resemble poison. Yoga poses may seem like poison at first, but in my experience, as time and practice continue, they become more like heaven.

Balance and Symmetry

I have always wondered whether Aristotle read and was influenced by early yogic texts when he invented the Golden Mean. The ancient ideals of balance and symmetry are basic to yoga, and like Aristotle's Golden Mean, not too little and not too much, should inform your practice.

This idea of moderation, of taking the middle road, of balance and symmetry applies to you as you begin to do yoga to relieve your back pain. Begin there, and you are likely to enjoy yoga and unlikely to hurt yourself. There are forms of yoga that I don't like, because they are too vigorous. They stress the physical aspect of the practice and neglect the rational. In order to progress you need a balance between the physical and the mental. When doing each pose in this book, you need to use your own discretion and discrimination. Don't rush headlong into any one pose. Be aware of contrasts, for example: flexibility/strength, mind/body, feelings/thoughts. In each of these pairs the apparent opposites are closely linked in human life. Strength alone can provide the stability to generate and endure stretching; conscious, intelligent work with your body will produce desirable results in your mind; quieting thoughts allow feelings to emerge; and so on. All of these apply to what you will be doing. In your practice, remember both sides of the coin.

Almost a direct extension of balance is symmetry. In most structures, whether they are animal, vegetable, or mineral, or whether they are constructions we have made, the rule is that more symmetrical is more balanced. Of course that's true of our bodies. We're symmetrical in the right to left plane, though not in the front to back plane or top to bottom. That one plane, however, has a great deal to do with balance. Yoga takes this into consideration, pursuing the Golden Mean by instructing that any pose that is done on the right side must also be done on the left. Please abide by this cardinal rule: If you have done it on one side, do not neglect the other side. Forgetting often enough to repeat on the left what you have done on the right opens you to injury, to unflattering and possibly harmful overdevelopment of one side, to loss of balance.

When it comes to actually doing the yoga, pursuing balance and symmetry will take you a long way.

Pushing Yourself

Should you push yourself? If so, how hard? Should you stop doing yoga the moment you feel the slightest twinge? Should yoga be entirely painless? These are questions that come up for everyone who has back pain, no matter what its source.

Again, I urge that you select the poses that are suggested for your own individual type of back pain. If you don't know what's causing your back pain, get a professional diagnosis. In ancient times, some yogis made extravagant claims: for example, "This pose banishes death," or "That pose causes the gastric fires to rage." At this point, because of our knowledge of human anatomy, we know that there are definite causes, definite effects, and definite cures for back pain.

After you have identified those poses most likely to help you, I advise "flirting" with them for a week or two before "embracing" them. In other words, you should do these poses once or at most twice a day for ten to fifteen seconds each, and with mild to moderate intensity. Eventually, through trial and observation, you will find a group of poses that help. Please note that all the poses in this book can be considered safe, but do not do any yoga pose in the following pages without reading the cautions. And start with the modified versions. Almost without exception, they're safer and easier than the regular poses. Exceptions are noted. Each chapter begins with poses appropriate for acute pain and moves to poses suitable for helping more chronic pain.

The first time you try a pose, I would say, don't stretch a muscle. Just practice as if it were a dress rehearsal rather than a performance, or like shadowboxing where no one gets hit. Just see what it would feel like to try that specific pose. If your pain doesn't worsen, if you have no significant ill effects, then you can embark on doing a specific pose more often and more energetically. Do this gradually. I would say 10 percent of what you imagine you should be doing is what you should do the first day. The second day I wouldn't increase it at all. Patience is a great virtue, a great form of self-discipline. I'm afraid it's the first thing you have to develop if you want to do yoga properly.

If you have a teacher, you can listen to the teacher's guidance, and that is better than just reading it in a book. However, if for one reason or another you're just reading about a pose, you may increase the level of your exertion and stretch by 10 percent a week, so that in ten weeks you'll be doing the best you can. Once you have reached 100 percent of your capacity, you will find that you keep advancing beyond what it seemed possible that you could do. I have found during the many years I have practiced yoga that the poses promote their own perfection, but after thirty years I am still on the way to perfection. With practice you will begin to notice that different poses have different effects on your back pain. By being alert and acting in your own behalf, you'll soon be able to select a series of yoga poses that will aid you more and more.

Some of the poses will "work" right away, after you come out of the pose, or even while you're in it. Others increase range of motion of nearby joints, lessening the strain on the troubled region. They may take weeks or months to be effective. But they not only relieve pain; they also go some distance toward preventing recurrence. Begin, however, with the poses in the chapter or chapters that correspond to your needs. Do the poses in the order in which they appear. If necessary, you can later make additions, subtractions, or adjustments.

Patting Your Head, Rubbing Your Stomach

Some people are a little intimidated when they contemplate assuming a complicated yoga pose, or any yoga pose at all. To those individuals I say, the proper approach to a yoga pose is to divide and conquer. If there are five steps to the pose and you can't do them all singly, let alone together, begin with one—the simplest. Do that. Then add another element of the pose. Slowly, slowly put those two together and add a third one. Keep going.

Which Poses?

I have advised you to find out what type of back pain you have and then to do the poses I have specifically chosen to relieve it. However, people who have one form of back pain will frequently benefit from poses that are not specifically oriented toward their back pain but toward a similar problem.

Suppose you have sacroiliac joint derangement, which is a painful condition that occurs when the sacroiliac joints are not completely aligned. Your pain is being relieved pretty consistently and well as you do the poses in that chapter. If that's the case, then you might want to try looking at the poses for piriformis syndrome because those will stretch the muscles in an ever-greater radius around the points that trouble you. After that, it could be helpful to try the poses for musculoskeletal pain. And so on. The poses in this book can be considered a basis for a yoga practice. These poses are not just good for back pain; they have many other advantages. The converse is also true. They may not be good for your back pain, but they may be good for you

How Long the Pose, How Long the Yoga

When it comes to the length of time you should spend doing any one pose, it's the same divide-and-conquer technique. I have heard that there are teachers in Tibet who demand of their students that they find a pose and then work to stay in that pose for three hours. One person tried to do this with headstand. Here's the way he accomplished the task. First he did the pose for five minutes, then ten minutes, and finally for twenty minutes. When he could reliably do it for twenty minutes, he planned to do the pose once, then rest for twenty minutes, and after that break do the pose for twenty minutes again. Gradually, minute by minute, he shortened the time between the two repetitions of the pose until he was doing it not twice for twenty minutes as he did at the beginning, but he was doing it just once for forty minutes. Then he did it again with two forty-minute sessions, and then again with eighty-minute sessions. I believe that technique is one secret of increasing your time in a pose.

But the opposite approach is also very effective. Do every pose once, then stop. Be satisfied with having done a sequence of poses a single, good time. If you have back pain, if your back pain is laying you up and you have nothing else to do, you can work with, and experiment with, a number of yoga poses during the day. You might find one pose where even the flirtation does you some good.

At first I would say it's more important to pay attention to what you're doing than to how long a time or how short a time you're spending. When all is said and done, if you're not spending between ten and twenty minutes a day at least experimenting with the poses, then you may be wasting your time. Keep in mind that the attitude and mood with which you approach yoga are very important.

Getting In and Getting Out

There is a specific way to enter a yoga pose and a specific way to leave it. When you begin, you need to build up a series of movements that become smoother as you enter the correct position. The sequence of movements that takes you into an unfamiliar position has a particular order, and it is a good idea to follow it to avoid making errors that lead to injury or making the pose less effective. The same holds true when you are coming out of a pose. If you've never done it, it's important that you do it right. If you're already doing it, check it out just the same. You don't necessarily come out of a pose in exactly the opposite way you went in. In other words, if you have a map of the way to get from here to Harry's house, you would think you would have a map of how to get from Harry's house back to your home. That doesn't hold for all these yoga poses, because gravity sometimes intervenes, and gravity is a one-way street. A good example of this is the headstand (see page 143). Since there is no universal rule, it is best to learn the way to get into each pose and the way to get out of it.

Remember, yoga is not just calisthenics. Yoga is a specifically designed program to use your body to control your mind and use your mind to control your body; it is meant to increase strength and coordination, to get relaxed, to court symmetry, to work on stretching muscles, extending capacities, and being able to do new things. In order to pursue it properly, following instructions is critical. Hopefully, following instructions will instill in you a sense of the symmetry, calm, balance, and relaxation that are intrinsic in yoga and critical to eliminating your back pain.

Inhaling and Exhaling

If you try to hold your breath for long, signals coming from your hypothalamus and brain stem will stimulate you to start breathing again. You can fight these urges and continue trying to hold your breath, but the impulses are still there, unless you hold your breath long enough to pass out. When that happens, autonomic functions will take over again and your breathing will continue at the rate your nervous system dictates.

Your breath and heartbeat represent the only two things that you sense your body must do with a certain given regularity. Actually your blood is circulating, your intestines are digesting, and under the surface the rest of the body is also very busy. Some few and exceptional yogis have learned to control their heart rate, but you (and everyone else) can regulate the speed at which you breathe, at least to some extent. Let me make two analogies: Your muscles have a given maximum strength at any given time, but yoga can help you change that, making muscles stronger and more flexible through voluntary intervention. In the same way, by learning to control the rate and intensity with which you draw in and expel air, yoga may help you accomplish certain goals, such as becoming calmer and more focused. Through voluntary intervention, you can increase your range of motion and extend the limits of your joints; this in turn expands the activities you can pursue without developing back pain.

When you breathe in, the muscles of your ribs contract to hold the ribs apart like the staves of a barrel. Your diaphragm descends, so that a partial vacuum is created. Lower pressure in the chest works to draw air in and to draw blood in from other parts of the body. This changes the way your heart contracts and relaxes, as it does with every beat. Your heart relaxes more easily with lower pressure in your chest. Conversely, when you are breathing out you put more pressure on your chest and your heart will eject blood more forcibly.

The same is true of the blood vessels of your chest. Just as air does, more blood will rush in when you're breathing in and more blood will be pressed out when you're exhaling. You should breathe calmly at all times in your life, but when you're doing yoga you can control it and focus on it.

Breathing also affects an elemental membrane inside you, a fascial layer that starts down at your buttocks and extends up into your skull and down into your legs. This fascia lines your whole body above and below the muscles, but also inside your chest and outside your abdominal organs and lungs. It anchors your heart. While this layer of membranous tissue moves a great deal when you move, the paradox is that it also restricts movement because it is connective tissue and contains no muscles itself.

Muscles attached all the way up and down the fascia, from your neck and shoulders to your groin, can stretch.[1] That's one of the things that happens when you do yoga. In addition, when you're breathing in and out, this fascia changes shape, like a balloon being squeezed. These changes affect your heart, your liver, and all the rest of your internal organs.

Finding a Teacher, Class, or Therapist/Teacher

Even the best private schools sometimes have poor teachers. If you have back pain what you need is individual attention, at least at first. Probably the best you could do would be to find a physician who is a yogi. Second best would be to find a physician who is familiar with yoga, yoga therapists, and yoga teachers.

There is a distinction between a teacher of yoga and a person who uses yoga in therapy, though some schools or styles are more useful for therapy than others. A yoga therapist is what you are seeking. There is a group of these therapists, called the International Society of Yoga Therapists. But probably not everyone who is a capable yoga therapist is in this group. Conversely, there may be people in this society who are not suitable for your individual needs.

A personal trainer, a private yoga teacher, or a coach is somewhere between a teacher and a therapist. It is probably wise to gravitate toward a teacher/therapist with at least five to ten years of experience in using hatha yoga as therapy. If you cannot locate an MD who is also a yoga therapist, you may be able to find an osteopath, a physical or occupational therapist, a nurse, or a chiropractor who can guide you.

Whomever you choose, that person should have anatomical knowledge—familiarity with muscles and other tissues, organ systems, and physiology. Knowledge of kinesiology—how contraction/relaxation of muscles translates into movement, dysfunction, and pain—is also fundamental. It is also crucial that your teacher/therapist talk to you before you begin practicing. You need an idea of what's wrong and a plan for solving your problem or problems. Your teacher should be gentle, should be willing to talk and to listen, and should demonstrate flexibility in adjusting your practice in a nonformulaic way over time.

Your back pain entitles you to be extra careful in choosing a teacher. Not all will be equally understanding, knowledgeable, competent, or sympathetic. You want to find somebody dedicated to therapeutic yoga, healing through yoga, not just yoga.

There are a number of schools of yoga, some probably more effective than others. Having studied with B.K.S. Iyengar, I regard the Iyengar school as being the most psychologically erudite and therapeutically oriented. Anusara is also an excellent method, as is the Integral yoga approach. My next choice would be a teacher/therapist who is eclectic—someone who does a little of this and a little of that, but is suited to what you want and need. Ignorance may masquerade under the banner of eclecticism, but this approach can be the real thing too.

Finally, have your physician and your yoga teacher communicate if possible. At least have your physician write down a detailed diagnosis you can show your yoga instructor. Your yoga therapist/teacher should know when the oversight of a medical professional is needed. This book should help you know that, too.

Reasons to see a health professional include: continuing pain for two weeks, reduced control of bowel or bladder, increasing weakness in lower extremities, numbness that ascends from feet toward knees, extreme pain, inability to stand, walk, or work.

Where and What to Wear

Where should you do yoga? The answer is anywhere you have a clean, quiet space that is big enough. I spread out a mat in my living room and do my yoga there every morning before the rest of the household is awake so that I have a calm basis for my practice. By the way, I don't use that mat for anything other than yoga.

I wear a pair of gym shorts and an ordinary T-shirt and do yoga in bare feet. Your clothes should be clean and comfortable, neither too big and blousy nor too small and tight. As far as I'm concerned, style is unimportant.

However, sometimes you need to do yoga or meditate in stressful situations. When that happens, you can adapt in many ways. For example, you can do both physical yoga and meditation in other kinds of places: on an airplane, in the backseat of a car, while riding the subway.

Props

You can almost always find props you need around the house—a chair, a cushion, a bed pillow, a belt, a thick book. There are also inexpensive aids you can buy at sporting-goods stores, health clubs, and on the Internet. These include blocks, yoga straps, and card-table chairs that are specially designed with adequate space between the seats and backs for doing yoga.

CHAPTER 4

Pain

What is pain? We know it when we feel it, but it's not so easy to put into words. In 1979 the taxonomy committee of the International Association of the Study of Pain was able to come up with a definition, which still has relevance. "[Pain] is an unpleasant sensory and emotional experience associated with actual or potential tissue damage, or described in terms of such damage," the committee stated. "Pain is always subjective." With those last few words, the committee added a crucial element.

What makes telling anyone about the pain you feel so difficult is precisely its subjective nature. The philosopher Ludwig Wittgenstein said, "I cannot feel your pain." Any pain the philosopher felt was his own. That's the human condition. Nobody can feel your pain; you can't feel anyone's pain. All you can do is empathize. A physician like myself, looking at a patient's MRI, may see a herniated disc of the sort that sometimes hurts terribly. Yet the patient may insist she feels nothing. Her truth must become mine. Of course, the opposite situation may also exist, when a patient feels tremendous pain for which I can find no apparent reason.

Symptoms and Signs

Symptoms are the unpleasant physical problems that usually bring patients to doctors, who then make a diagnosis and prescribe treatment. Anything you feel subjectively and must communicate to another person in words is a symptom. That means pain, heaviness, tingling, ache, or any one of a number of other types of discomfort. You are the only one who knows where and how much it hurts and the only one who can express all that in words. You're the world's expert on your own pain.

Signs are the external manifestations of illness and injury. A fever is a sign, but dizziness, blurry vision, cramps, earache, stiffness, a feeling of being "chilly" are symptoms. Swelling is a sign. Signs are the opposite of symptoms, because they're objective. Nausea is a symptom; vomiting is a sign. A keen observer, your health-care worker may tap on your knees to check your reflexes, may press on a muscle to see how tight it is, may listen to your heartbeat. A sign is also the result of a diagnostic test performed with equipment—the number on a blood test, the contents of a spinal tap, what an imaging study like an X ray or an MRI tells the doctor.

The distinction between symptoms and signs is an important one for helping you understand your conversations with your doctor, and for communicating with your yoga teacher. The trained interpretation of symptoms and signs in the context of a medical history is what clinicians call a medical exam. This involves the Review of Systems: a checklist of symptoms and signs created by great Greek, Arabian, and Jewish physicians of the Middle Ages and earlier, which every contemporary medical student must memorize. The medical exam encapsulates wisdom gathered by many healers over the millennia, and some say it accounts for 90 percent of the conclusions that comprise a diagnosis.

Intensity

If your pain interrupts your concentration and daily activities or makes it difficult to work, enjoy your leisure time, or sleep, it's time, or past time, to do something about it. If you would describe your pain as slight or moderate, you may not need to see a health-care worker, unless it persists for more than two weeks. A dull, persistent ache that goes on and on can exhaust and depress you. Get help if you have symptoms for more than fourteen days.

There are scales your doctor may use to help you gauge the severity of your pain. These scales have been used with some success to quantify pain, to make a reliable, objective correlate. These scales ask you to "grade" your pain on a scale of one to ten, or they present a drawing of a person, front and back, and ask the patient to use multiple-choice descriptions of where and how much it hurts.

A pain scale is useful in gauging the effectiveness of physical therapy, acupuncture, medicines, and exercise like yoga. You might find it an interesting exercise to assign your pain a number from one to ten and to make a note of the number several times a week to see if yoga is making a difference for you.

> 0—no pain at all
> 2—bearable pain anyone might experience from carrying a
>   heavy bundle too far or standing on one's feet too long
> 5—pain that often interferes with your concentration
> 7—intense pain that takes the pleasure out of daily activities
>   and is the chief focus of your attention most of the time
> 9—pain that may make you feel like screaming
> 10—unbearable pain, a medical emergency

Some people find it difficult to locate pain with any certainty. It seems to move from place to place. Others have trouble finding the words to describe their pain. The McGill-Melzack Pain Questionnaire, popular with physicians, has more than seventy-five words to describe pain, including *flickering, jumping, pricking, lacerating, pinching, gnawing, cramping, scalding, itchy, sore, heavy, taut, tiring, sickening, annoying, spreading, nagging,* and *dreadful.*

Time spent finding the proper words to describe and locate your pain is not wasted. As Wittgenstein asked, "How could I get between a man and his pain?" Words are insubstantial enough to do just that.

Acute and Chronic Pain

The way you approach yoga is determined in some measure by whether your pain is chronic or acute and, of course, by your underlying physical condition. Assume for a minute that your pain is chronic. Let's say it comes and goes, that it hampers you but doesn't cripple you. You don't play tennis the way you used to; you don't jog. But you can go on with your life. If this describes the type of pain you have, then yoga is exactly the right thing for you. You should start slowly. Get a diagnosis, then find the poses that are appropriate and helpful for you, and go straight ahead.

If your pain is acute, yoga may also be for you but you are going to have to proceed a little differently. You will need to be mindful of the pain itself. It's not the chronic condition that is your target here; it's the pain you're experiencing while you are actually doing the yoga poses. I'm making a distinction between doing the poses so you won't feel pain (chronic) and doing the poses so you will relieve the pain you already feel (acute). In the second case the disadvantage is that the pain itself can keep you from doing too much yoga. But the advantage is that you can actually feel the effect of the pose as you do it. You have instant feedback on your pain. If doing a specific pose or a number of poses makes your pain worse, don't continue. However, it is worth talking to someone with adequate experience and knowledge who can give you advice before ceasing all activity. There are many kinds of pain that we all know about that get worse before they get better.

You may be experiencing that type of pain. A tight hamstring has to stretch. That's something that isn't painful to start with, but when you make it hurt a little, you know very well what you're doing. A hamstring that's in spasm is extremely painful, and unfortunately the only way to relieve it is to stretch it. That often produces significantly more pain before you get the benefit of relief. That's the type of additional pain that should not deter you. On the other side of the increased pain that comes with the stretch is the diminution of the discomfort.

If you feel a sharp, tingling, or stabbing pain while doing yoga, stop what you are doing immediately! This is especially true if you are pregnant. The type of pain that comes from slowly stretching muscles, ligaments, joint capsules, or fascia is the only type of pain that is acceptable.

Do not do the stretch or the pose that is to relieve a spasm unless you can identify the spasm. When you can feel that the muscle is tight, when pressing on it relieves pain, when you can see muscle contraction, then stretch can be a good thing. If you have a pinched nerve, that very same pose you found helped you with a muscle spasm can hurt you instead.

If you have sacroiliac joint derangement, you may need to stretch the muscles around the joint a little. A little pain may bring relief later if you have arthritis. To relieve the dull, aching pain of piriformis syndrome, you will need to cause yourself a little bit more pain, since this problem is usually associated with muscle spasm as well as a nerve compressed by the tightened muscle. If you have spinal stenosis, the acceptable stretch is in the muscles, nowhere else. The red stoplight goes on if you feel any stinging, numbing, or other neurological symptoms.

Muscular Pain

"Nonspecific backache" is the fifth most common reason patients visit doctors. Included in this diagnosis are muscle spasms, sprains, strains, sacroiliac joint pain, and backache caused by nonneurological conditions, stress, and other emotional problems.

If you feel a dull, manageable ache in the area of your lower back, you probably have musculoskeletal pain. It is possible to verify this by placing your thumbs a little above your waist, three or four inches to either side of your spine. If pressing on the muscles there—the quadratus lumborum and the serratus inferior posterior—produces pain, it may be that you have lifted something too heavy or worked too hard in the garden.

Try putting your hands on your hips and "walking" upward with your thumbs. When you can feel the curves of your ribs, you may feel pain. The problem could have come from twisting or moving from side to side while carrying something heavy, like a suitcase, from parking a van without power steering, or from an awkward repetitive movement.

Neurological Pain

Tip-offs:
- If your pain follows the pattern of nerves in your body, i.e., sciatica, where pain descends to the thigh, calf, and/or foot
- If your muscles don't ache but do feel stiff
- If you have distinctive pain, for example feelings of electrical shock

People who have back problems often suffer from neuropathic pain. In a sense, all pain (and pleasure) is neurological since the nervous system participates in anything we feel. Neuropathic pain arises not only when the nervous system communicates and registers the pain, but also when the pain originates from damage or other causes that affect the nervous system itself.

Diabetes mellitus, for example, can cause unpleasant tightening of the shoulder capsule, the discomfort of which is communicated to the pain centers in the brain through the nervous system. This is not neuropathic pain. However, the elevated blood sugar seen in diabetes can also cause direct damage to neurons, giving rise to painful sensations of burning, tightness, and tingling, which would be classified as neuropathic pain. The injury to neurons caused by increased concentration of blood sugar can also cause numbness. That scenario gives rise to a strange possibility: The injured neurons might actually reduce the pain coming from a non-neurological cause—in this case, a painful shoulder. In other words, a person with a frozen shoulder and a neuropathy caused by diabetes might not feel the pain of the shoulder condition because pain-communicating neurons don't function properly.

I have seen this situation. Generally it results in gross damage to the joint, since the patient is getting no feedback that draws attention to the orthopedic condition. This phenomenon—when you don't feel what ought to hurt—also applies to low back pain.

The injury that causes pain in the low back can also reduce the ability of the spinal cord to carry signals up and back from the point of injury to the brain. In a sense this may muffle your body's call for help, reducing awareness of the condition that is causing harm.

When reflexes are working normally, a tap on the knee activates the sensory nerve, bringing impulses up to your spinal cord, where they synapse with a motor neuron to make the muscle move. If you have an injury in your spinal cord, it's quite possible that it will interfere with the nerve conduction and, finally, the reflex. The most serious injury of this sort occurs when there is an injury in the lower back, which can interfere with the sensory nerves that carry feelings of fullness from the bowel and bladder, affecting control. Also the sphincters of the bowel and bladder may not work properly because the motor neurons that actually keep them closed aren't working, or because the brain isn't functioning the way it should.

Neurological problems can also affect your locomotion. The way you walk, your gait, is a delicate process that depends on coordination of an extensive pattern of signals that go up from the bottom of your foot to your knee and hip when you move your leg forward. The nerve impulses direct the movement of your leg until you finally put your foot down in front of you to begin the next step. If your gait becomes abnormal, for example with "dropped" foot, you could have problems with the motor system or the sensory system or a combination of the two. If this happens, obviously the danger of falling is greatly increased.

Danger signals: Go to the emergency room immediately if you are actually weak, if numbness ascends your legs, or if you lose control of your bowels or bladder. These symptoms and signs could signal that the nerves ascending in the spinal cord are being compressed to the point where they may actually die, causing permanent disability. While neurological pain may be intense, all high-level pain is not neurological. Do not try to ignore any pain that approaches the unbearable or excruciating; it should be promptly diagnosed by a competent medical professional.

Sometimes symptoms and signs are localized, existing in a particular part of the body. For example, the feeling of tightness you get when you have sunburn is a symptom you can easily "place" in the skin. That is opposed to the redness the sun may produce, which is an objectively observable sign. But nerves are everywhere. Blushing, even though it may be due to something subjective, is, after all, objective and observable. If we consider the endocrine system, then if someone feels hot and has a rapid heart rate, the sensation of heat is a symptom and the heart rate is a sign of hyperthyroidism. The nervous system, however, is the largest system in the body to which symptoms and signs are ascribed. That's natural. The nervous system is the foundation of behavior and feelings, and in any movement, it's part of the act.

Pain with Specific Activities

With neurological pain there is a classical, structural approach to finding the cause. Damage to individual anatomical elements results in signs and symptoms. For example, the MRI may locate a specific spot where a nerve root is compressed by a herniated disc. The clinician knows that particular nerve root supplies the skin at the inner calf and the muscles that raise the foot at the ankle. If the patient slaps that foot on the floor and complains of tingling and numbness above the ankle when walking, the physician can make a diagnosis before a word is spoken.

In cases where there is neurological pain, however, there may also be problems with the integration and coordination of the anatomical elements. It may not be possible to isolate a particular pathology of any kind. Piece by piece, the anatomy is just fine but the situation as a whole may be like a dysfunctional family of four healthy, basically happy people who come together and make each other miserable. For instance, a somewhat overweight flight attendant with mildly narrowed nerve openings in the spine may arch his back just enough when leaning over to serve the person in the window seat to cause electric shocks along the femoral nerve in the leg.

But of course other problems may also cause pain. You can have another dysfunctional family consisting not of nerves, but of muscles, bones, and joints. The history teacher whose posture is somewhat hunched over but in the normal range who also has a slightly backward-tilted sacroiliac joint may have terrific back pain throughout the school day. And if you have two perfectly normal legs that just happen to be of slightly different lengths, you may have a different but also painful problem.

I have a vigorous patient, an older man who lives at the shore. In the summer he likes to exercise by walking through chest-high seawater. This gentleman came to me because of a puzzling situation.

He had terrific pain when he walked east through the water and felt fine when he walked west. Finding that this man has a leg length discrepancy solved the problem. When he walked with the long leg closer to the shoreline, the slope of the beach added to the difference in the lengths of his legs. It was as if he were walking with one foot on the street and the other on a high curb. Walking in the opposite direction the slope of the ocean floor made up for the discrepancy in the length of his legs.

Actually, there are five ways that doing a specific activity can cause pain:

- You're doing it incorrectly.
- Individual muscles or muscle groups aren't equipped for the task.
- There's an anatomical mismatch that causes damage or pain.
- Poor approach.
- You're doing it for too long.

In the case of a mismatch, take the yoga pose called Marichyasana. If you have stubby arms and a prominent abdomen, trying to place your arms behind your back and then clasping your hands will be either impossible, or possible at the price of moving something farther than it ought to go. If you feel that your body parts are not meant to or can't perform a certain activity, common sense and reason ought to come in and take the place of enthusiasm.

Poor approach is often linked with poor posture. At work your chair may be too low. Holding your elbow out while typing might have a negative effect anywhere along your back. If you lean forward squinting at a computer screen for too long, you may cause yourself pain. In my experience people who do physical work may overdo it, but those who have white-collar jobs are at risk for the same mistake.

Yoga may be a specific activity that causes pain. The BBC News has reported that doctors and physiotherapists have observed a surge in the number of inexperienced student yogis hurting themselves after doing difficult or unfamiliar asanas.[1] According to this report, the most frequent injuries are those that come from repetitive strain or overstretching, and the wrists, shoulders, neck, spine, sacroiliac joint, hamstrings, and knees are the most vulnerable. Avoid injury by making sure your teacher has adequate training and realize that the cautions above apply.

Yoga may also be used as an analytical tool to diagnose pain caused by another activity. If you find that certain yoga poses or elements of them are hurting, you should discuss it with someone skilled at both yoga and diagnosis. Your doctor or teacher/therapist may be able to use the pose as a way of figuring out what's wrong.

What you do away from work is, of course, easier to change and adjust than what you must do while you earn a living. However, to quote an old saying: "Don't let your work interfere with your fishing." For many, giving up beloved leisure activities is simply not an option. If that's true for you, and if those out-of-work pastimes are causing physical discomfort, search for ways to make accommodations.

When Yoga Is Not Enough

Every therapy has its limitations. It may be difficult to identify when it is time to move on, with or without yoga, but definitely to take some additional measures to control pain and cure the problem that is causing it. Three such criteria are:

- When you get disabled from doing something such as driving, working, walking, or doing anything that is important for you to do.
- When it hurts or tingles enough to disturb your concentration, whether it's working, cooking, shopping, watching a movie, talking, reading, etc.
- When compensation for it starts causing other things to happen that aren't readily controlled: in order for the hip to behave, you start walking or sleeping a little differently, which makes the upper back hurt. If you change your posture ever so slightly, and then your neck ends up stiff, you might take one more Motrin, but the stomach wishes you hadn't.

It's All in Your Head

Some individuals spend years trudging from doctor to doctor, explaining their pain as well as they can. Although their pain is real, they may not find a physician clever enough to make a diagnosis and prescribe an effective treatment. In some cases it may seem impossible to find a viable diagnosis.

Usually, when a doctor looks at you and says, "It's all in your head, dear," it's a condescending and disrespectful way to say that you don't seem to have any of the five or six major causes of back pain, and therefore there is no cause at all. As far as I'm concerned, if this happens to you, you should thank that doctor and then walk out and look for a diagnostician capable of finding out what's wrong. You may very well have one of the problems the doctor has dismissed, or any number of "composite" causes, such as the ones discussed above.

There's no question that Freud was onto something real when he spoke of the "Conversion Syndrome," meaning the transformation of a mental state or problem into a physical one. But in twenty-five years of medical practice, I have not seen this as the full explanation for any patient's pain. Nevertheless, there are ways where pain is magnified or diminished quite consciously or not quite consciously.

- Identification
- Focus
- Feedback

If you are a kid sleeping out in a tent with your friends for the first time, and they start screaming about a spider infestation, you might identify the normal movement of your pajama leg caused by your own squirming as a spider coming to bite you. If you had a muscle spasm in your back a year ago, you might fear and even begin to believe a much less serious muscular problem is a new spasm. Identification may heighten anxiety, tighten muscles, and actually produce the thing you're guarding against. This is particularly true with feared diseases. A patient once said to me, "Doctor, I only feel the pain when I start thinking I might have cancer."

Then there is the incident that makes you focus on pain or the possibility of it. Say someone just coasting along in his car bumps into the back of your car, and for the rest of the day all you can think about is the pain you might get. After a while you begin to feel a little something in your neck, and then in your shoulder. Unconsciously you stiffen your neck and shoulder, tighten the muscles, and change the blood supply to those muscles, increasing the chances that your mental state may cause physical discomfort.

Or it's feedback. When a car going three miles an hour bumps yours, you may focus on the possibility of pain. Your face takes on an expression of concern, of unhappy expectation. Several studies have documented that if you simply make a face, put on an expression of sadness or disgust, you may actually feel sadness or disgust. Or in the case of the small automobile accident, your facial expression afterwards as you think about what happened could suggest that your brain sent you a message that you are beginning to feel some pain.[2]

I've had a desperate patient say to me, "What can I do if it's all in my head?" Having a backache makes some people feel guilty, especially if there's no dramatic explanation, such as a fracture or a herniated disc. But now we know that a person's low back pain may be related to stress, anxiety, or a number of other psychological factors. Dr. John Sarno, Professor of Rehabilitation at New York University's School of Medicine and attending physician at the Howard A. Rusk Institute of Rehabilitation, has been a leading figure in helping patients work on stress, which results in low back pain, which results in more stress.[3]

Stress is a well-documented factor in low back pain. A recent study conducted in the Department of Environmental Health at the University of Cincinnati won the Volvo Award in Biomechanics. Investigators gave individual participants heavy boxes to lift and simple or complex decisions to make. The study concluded that mental stress could result in less controlled movements and increases in trunk muscle coactivation—physical adjustments that raise the risk of low back pain.[4]

Ernest Holmes, author of *The Science of Mind*, and Dr. Harold Koenig, author of *The Healing Power of Faith* and other books, Larry Dossey, author of *Prayer Is Good Medicine*, and many others have turned to religion for ways to deal with pain. These advocates assert that prayer can actually modulate pain and illness, possibly by reducing stress.[5]

Last, there is another type of focus—positive focus. Your back may hurt, but if you are able to put your focus elsewhere, you may be able to go on with your day more constructively. I think of the memorial monument of the American fighters raising the flag on Iwo Jima during World War II. Some had injuries; others had even been shot. They were smiling anyway. They weren't paying attention to what was hurting, but were focusing on something that gave them pride and satisfaction. That all but made the pain seem as if it had been all in their heads.

CHAPTER 5

Major Causes of Low Back Pain

Whether it's yoga, physical therapy, over-the-counter painkillers, environmental changes, injections of anesthetics and/or other substances, or undergoing a surgical procedure, there is a solution for most low back pain. I admit that for some people the right treatment isn't so easy to find. That's because so much of lower back pain is undiagnosed. Many patients who come to me have previously seen a number of other doctors and therapists without finding relief. Some of these patients are depressed, and some have almost lost hope.

I say to these discouraged individuals and to anyone else suffering from chronic low back pain that the cure is often a piece of cake—if and only if you know your diagnosis. Without knowing the source of your problem, or problems, how can you find the right way to go about solving it? I mention problems in the plural because sometimes individuals know they are in pain but are not aware that they can also have what I jokingly call "fleas and lice." What I mean is that a person with sacroiliac joint derangement may very well also have piriformis syndrome, or that leg length discrepancy can cause musculoskeletal problems. You may be someone whose diagnosis includes more than one major cause of low back pain.

Clearly, some people's pain calls for a physician's attention, for professionally administered diagnostic tests, for prescription medications, for physical therapy and other measures. These medical approaches and yoga are not mutually exclusive. In other words, having a problem that yields to medical treatment does not rule out your ability to help yourself by doing yoga. For some who are in acute pain and undergoing treatment, yoga breathing and meditation can be a godsend while the diagnostic and therapeutic processes take place.

If you don't know what's wrong, you can go some distance to understanding your own pain by yourself before embarking on a full medical investigation. Nor is it always necessary to wait for an official diagnosis before beginning yoga exercises. However, if your pain has been going on for more than two weeks, if there is progressive numbness in your feet, legs, or pelvic region or you are experiencing changes in bowel or bladder function, or if the pain is at a level you would describe as close to unbearable, seek medical advice before doing any type of physical exercise. As a general rule, I also emphasize that if doing physical yoga produces any type of neurological symptom—numbness, shooting or stabbing pain, tingling, or subsequent weakness—stop doing the pose immediately.

There is musculoskeletal pain, which is often associated with a specific activity, mood, or even a new pair of shoes. If your pain worsens for two or three days and then lessens, it may be that it is musculoskeletal, and yoga will do you good. It bears repeating that shooting pains, numbness, weakness, tingling, and strange sensations are linked with neurological pain, which can have more than one cause. These feelings are red flags. If you experience one or more of them, stop the activity and consult a physician before continuing. It's important, before pushing yourself in yoga or any other physical exercise, to be aware of the nature of your problem so you don't exacerbate it. But that doesn't mean that yoga won't help. The odds are high that it will. But in the strange land of severe pain, don't travel far without a diagnosis.

A fuller discussion of the major causes of low back pain I address in this book follows, but first, a note on weakness, a problem that crosses the entire spectrum of reasons people have back pain.

There may be two causes of weakness as it relates to back pain: neurological and musculoskeletal. The signals nerves bring of pressure, pain, temperature, and so on from your arms and legs back to your brain and the signals sent from your brain down to the muscles, blood vessels, and other structures of the arms and legs can be interrupted as they travel along their course. When these interruptions or disruptions take place, there are signs such as lack of sensation and reduction in muscle strength. This, of course, is weakness. Like numbness, weakness may be a symptom of nerve injury that can cause back pain. When an individual has back pain and weakness, sometimes a physician can learn the exact location of the problem along the course of a nerve from the pattern of the weakness in the body. This is weakness as a symptom of back pain.

However, there is something else to note here. Weakness, especially in the legs and in the extensor muscles of the spine, can be a cause of back pain apart from neurological problems. In that case the muscles are feeble, causing posture changes or compromises or adaptations that may bring the spine into a position that causes back pain. Actually this is the most common cause of back pain.

Musculoskeletal pain is frequently brought about by muscles that are too tight—exerting too strong a pull—or muscles that are too weak. Sometimes you can have a combination of the two. An example of that is the individual who has a pinched nerve in her back. Because of that, when she walks she cannot bring her foot up to swing it forward when the other foot is down. So she swings it out to the side and around in front of her, using other muscles that have not been disabled. To keep her balance she lurches subtly to the opposite side with every other step. This makes her change position in such a way that she develops a musculoskeletal problem in her back. Either the muscles that stabilize her spine ache from fatigue, or, if those muscles cease to stabilize the spine, vertebral joints may go out of alignment or develop arthritis. There the chief reason for the back pain is the adaptation, not the pinched nerve.

If you are experiencing weakness, please remember that it may be important—a reason to seek medical assistance. If the problem causing weakness is not systemic, then yoga will almost certainly be useful for helping an individual become stronger. An increase in strength is one of the main benefits of yoga. Some common causes of weakness are:

- Inactivity. This causes overall symmetrical weakness.
- Habitually sitting in chairs with too much support, slouching, reading propped up in bed, bending over for long periods of time may weaken extensor muscles that help arch the back.
- Joint derangement and osteoarthritis may activate inhibitory responses that effectively weaken the muscles around the joint.
- Surgery that cuts through muscles weakens them.

No matter why weakness has occurred, finding a way to combat it is essential, not only for the prevention and relief of back pain but for general physical well-being.

Weight Control

As we know, overweight is associated with diabetes, heart disease, respiratory difficulties, and a host of other problems. Many of us gain weight as we grow older, and those pounds, when carried around all the time in the course of daily life, may aggravate old injuries or cause new ones.

If you are pregnant, your doctor will give you an idea of optimal weight gain. For your own health and your baby's health, I hope you will follow those recommendations.

Even if you gain less weight than your doctor advises, however, you may be subject to back pain in the same way that overweight people are prone to it. Should back pain limit your feeling of well-being, discuss it with your doctor. Then try to find out whether this pain is musculoskeletal in origin or has some other cause. Chapter 13 should be helpful.

Weight gain if you are not pregnant is, of course, another matter. Finding out whether you're overweight isn't only a matter of consulting a chart based on gender and height, as it used to be. The government has added body mass to its calculation, along with something beautiful in its simplicity: waist circumference.

The National Center for Chronic Disease Prevention and Health

Promotion in the Centers for Disease Control recommends calculating your body mass index (BMI) to determine whether you need to lose weight.[1] You can use a calculator.

Divide your weight in pounds by the square of your height in inches. Multiply the result by 703. A person who is 5'7" tall and weighs 159 pounds has a BMI of 25. A 5'7" person who weighs 191 pounds has a BMI of 30. The range that is considered healthy is 19 to 25.

According to guidelines published by the NIH, a person with a BMI of 25 or greater is considered overweight; with a BMI of 30 or greater, the person is considered obese; and with a BMI of 40 or greater, the person is considered extremely obese. The BMI number applies to both men and women.

The next significant marker is waist circumference, which can be measured at the level of the navel or at the narrowest waist midpoint. A woman with a waist circumference over 35 inches or a man with a waist circumference over 40 inches should lose weight.

Musculoskeletal Pain

Musculoskeletal problems, including strains, sprains, spasm, and subluxation (which I will define and discuss shortly) and backache caused by stress and other emotional problems account for a great majority of low back pain.

How long this kind of pain lasts depends on your age, your general physical condition, the severity of the injury, the environment in which you live, and most important, what you do about it. Pain that is musculoskeletal in origin may disappear by itself after a period of time. It also responds well to over-the-counter painkillers, massage, and other noninvasive treatments like swimming. Yoga is an ideal way to deal with musculoskeletal low back pain, both acute and chronic.

Time is a significant factor in determining whether you have low back pain due to musculoskeletal problems. If you are in pain for more than two weeks, or if your pain is so acute you are having trouble participating in your regular work and leisure routines, then it may have a different cause; you should seek medical advice.

Posture

A pain in your neck, shoulders, ribs, and spine behind the ribs may come from the way you have adapted to a pain in your lower back. When both the lower and upper back hurt, the pain may have a single cause. That is, it is likely to be a result of a problem with posture. Adapting to the pain may have changed the way you stand and walk, brush your hair, bend to pick up a heavy package, or even the position in which you sleep at night.

The lumbar spine extending below the ribs to the coccyx (tailbone) is a weight-bearing structure, but it is relatively flexible, allowing for movement above the more or less fixed and weight-bearing pelvis. Muscles provide support for this part of the back, but its health and well-being are also contingent on an individual's strength, posture, coordination, and balance. The better these are, the more easily the lumbar spine can help balance weight, resist the pull of gravity, and withstand even greater stresses that movement places on its alignment and structures.

If your posture has changed because of a musculoskeletal injury or problem in the lumbar spine, there may be pain elsewhere. Correcting the original problem in the low back will make pain disappear all over.

Strain

When too much force is applied to the fibers that comprise muscles, ligaments, tendons, joint coverings, or even the joints themselves, these structures are pulled out of their proper alignment or formation. Celebrated physician of physical medicine and rehabilitation Renee Cailliet, in his book *Soft Tissue Pain and Disability*, describes situations that produce strain.[2] Here are the circumstances:

1. Undue force on a normal structure (i.e., lifting an object that is too heavy)
2. Normal force on an abnormally frail joint, muscle, tendon, or ligament

3. Normal stress on a normal but unprepared structure (shoveling snow for the first time in five years)
4. Performance of an awkward weight-bearing activity (lifting a box of books onto a high shelf)

Yoga poses that are excellent for strain include: Viparita Karani and Paschimottanasana, because in my experience these poses promote muscle relaxation and muscle relaxation allows for and leads to healing of strains.

Sprain

When strain goes a step further, muscle fibers, tendons, ligaments, or joint capsules may be pulled so far that some of them actually tear. Sprained structures often repair themselves over time, but not in every case. Since they heal slowly and because they are so painful, sprains can be more serious and difficult to deal with than fractures.

Gentle range-of-motion exercises, like Trikonasana and (for particularly stiff individuals) Dandasana, are yoga poses that may help if you have a hamstring sprain. If your problem is muscular, you can begin doing gentle yoga immediately. It will also reduce spasm.

Spasm

It happens when you're least expecting it. Suddenly something in your back clenches. It hurts! It's one muscle or it's a group of muscles in your back. They take over, and without conscious orders from you, they contract on their own. This intense, involuntary action causes what feels like an extreme cramp that can last a few seconds, a few minutes, or much longer.

A muscle in spasm is contracting, hard and involuntarily. It can happen in the back when you're gardening. It can happen in the thigh or the calf. A charley horse is a muscle spasm. This may be no laughing matter. A muscle spasm can last six months, or longer. This is a good example of why diagnosis is so important. For undiagnosed pain, two weeks is the limit before seeing a doctor. But once diagnosed, e.g., as a spasm, a long, gentle, self-administered course of yoga may be the safest and most effective treatment.

The tiny blood vessels that run through the muscle to nourish it and remove the waste products are squeezed during a muscle spasm, and therefore they have difficulty doing their job. Since blood flow is restricted, it cannot remove a typical, local, and temporary buildup of lactic acid. That causes the muscle to tighten further. The vicious cycle—spasm producing acids, acids increasing spasm—has begun, and may continue until the spasm becomes chronic.

Stretching is one of the most immediate, effective, and innocuous ways to interfere with that cycle of spasm, acid buildup, and more spasm. It is also a means of prevention of future spasm. All yoga poses involve stretching, but some are more suited to helping relieve spasm than others. If you think you have spasm in a muscle in your back, try doing Janusirsasana and Adho Mukha Svanasana. Use common sense when doing any yoga pose. Remember, yoga can add insult to injury if you stretch too much. Yoga should help you gain, not lose, control.

Subluxation and Dislocation

Soft tissues, muscles, sinews, and bands that connect and cover joints aren't the only possible problems: Sometimes the bones themselves are out of joint. When there is excessive or unusual pressure on a joint, one or more of the bones can slip out of their proper positions. A small amount of displacement is subluxation, or partial dislocation. It's dislocation when the surfaces are entirely separated.

The Emotional Component

As you probably already know, low levels of depression and high levels of stress can contribute to low back pain. Your problem may be as simple as a touch of Seasonal Affective Disorder (SAD) brought about by the cold, dark days of winter. It may be that you've started a new romance or moved your residence or changed jobs. Hatha (physical) yoga, breathing exercises, and meditation can be extremely effective in helping alleviate depression and in calming nervous tension due to stress. You are likely to feel a difference after just a few sessions.

Yoga is the only serious self-improvement program I know of that mandates: "Be contented" and "Be cheerful." This implies that mood is at least to some extent under a person's voluntary control. Dr. John Sarno, Dr. Harold Koenig, and Ernest Holmes, to name a few, have found effective ways to treat individuals by addressing anger, tension, pain, and even cognitive aspects of their personal lives. After all, these emotions and others are reflected in posture. You can see this for yourself just by looking in a full-length mirror. Yoga works not just on the physical and gross physiological features of the practitioner, but its goal is also spiritual. In my years as a practitioner of yoga and a doctor I have seen it significantly benefit emotions and mentality.

Herniated Vertebral Disc ("Pinched Nerve")

Horror stories abound about the pain of pinched nerves and herniated discs but actually these conditions account for only a little more than 10 percent of doctor visits for low back pain.[3] A herniated disc—also called a slipped disc or ruptured disc—always involves gelatinous disc material oozing out of the stiffer, fibrous covering of the one- to two-centimeter-high cylinder that separates the vertebral bones. This causes inflammation and swelling, which may compress a nerve or nerve roots at the spot where they emerge from the spinal column. What a pinched nerve and a "slipped," or herniated, disc have in common is that they cause all kinds of neurological symptoms, from a feeling of pins and needles to weakness, from severe pain to no feeling at all in the areas where that particular nerve's fibers end.

Something many patients don't know is that neurological pain can be referred. That means that it can originate anywhere along the spine, but it may be felt as far away as the big toe. If, while walking to the bathroom in the middle of the night, you stub your toe on a chair leg, you won't have any doubt about which foot—the left or the right—is affected. Nor will you wonder where the impact occurred. Because of the way our nerves work, what happens in the spine can be more complex. The point of the injury may be in your low back, but the damaged nerves may report painful sensation to the brain as coming from another place, far away from the spot where the injury occurred, for example to your outer left calf. If some of the fibers of the sciatic nerve are torn while exiting a specific part of the spine, for example, you may feel nothing there. Your back could be symptom-free, may feel so normal that it may even be hard to believe there could be an injury there. In this case, the pain or other unpleasant symptom will feel as if it's coming from the calf, because the brain misinterprets the signal as if it comes from the calf, where every previous signal those fibers carried has originated. You don't feel pain at the site of the injury. The cause of the pain is in the lumbar spine, but the manifestation is where the nerve endings lie, in the calf.

The word *sciatica* was coined in Renaissance Florence, where, of course, people also suffered from backache and from neurological symptoms originating in the back. The word *ischiatica* suggested the ischeal bones had a role in back pain. It was used because it was thought that sciatica came from tuberculosis involving the muscles near those bones. Now, of course, we know that sciatica can take many forms, and can originate in the back as a nerve root injury or in the piriformis muscle as compression of the same nerve fibers in the buttock. Similar pain may come from the sacroiliac joint in which case the pain rarely crosses the knee. It can change in type and location, can be intermittent or constant.

Sciatica is not a diagnosis. It's a symptom of a neurological problem somewhere along the anatomical length of the sciatic nerve. But sciatica has become a catch-all word to describe neurological symptoms that begin in the back and travel down the nerves into the lower extremities. These symptoms are many and varied. They include:

- Numbness, or a problem with nerve impulses traveling as they should, from skin to brain. Reduced or absent skin sensitivity usually occurs in legs and feet, and it may be hard to notice. Numbness is important, frequently providing a more reliable guide than pain for physicians seeking a diagnosis for back pain.
- Paraesthesias are strange sensations, including burning and tingling, and "crawling," which are due to abnormal signal patterns

reaching the brain. They are analogous to referred pain in that their point of causation is far from the site of the sensation. The strange sensations are located on the skin.

- Weakness (see above).
- Burning. Without clear and visible skin injury, a burning sensation may come from a pinched nerve root in the lumbar spine or a large peripheral nerve, resulting in mild to intolerable discomfort on the trunk, low back, buttocks, genital area, legs, and feet.
- Electric shock. This feeling is often caused by a structural problem like a radiculopathy (see below) and may occur at the moment the thousands of fibers that make up a nerve are compressed, causing them to discharge all at once. Sometimes electric shock–like pain is constant, but in each short burst there is a beginning, a middle, and an end. It also has a direction; for example, it may go from the buttock to the calf. This lightning-bolt type of pain may come and go with changes in position or pressure, for example when lifting heavy objects.

Arthritis

Osteoarthritis (degenerative joint disease). Normal wear and tear eventually leads to this form of arthritis for most of us. In addition, postural or other problems, or overuse, may hasten this painful condition of the joints. Why? An X ray or MRI of the hip joint shows nearly perfect spheres. The cartilage on the surface of the hip joint and the pelvis is made by cells in a similar arrangement underneath each half of the joint.

If the cartilage on the surface is injured, it's no big deal. Like a fingernail or a hair, it is replaced by the cells underneath. However, if the underlying cartilage is injured, two problems occur. One part of the joint surface becomes uneven, and then can rub against the other surface, injuring it. Deeper injury may deform the cells that actually produce the cartilage. As a result, the formation of the cartilage will be chronically irregular. The original smooth, spherical shape will be lost. Once this process begins, and it is inevitable for everyone, it goes further and further. One abnormal surface is sure to cause abnormalities in the other, which will soon return the favor.

Yoga appears to slow this process and to make the joints more functional.[4]

Yoga is beneficial for osteoarthritis, because it appears to stretch the joint capsules and the muscles around them—in the case of the spine, for example, the multifidus, iliocostalis, and quadratus lumborum muscles. Range of motion can be increased for restricted joints by doing yoga. It has been suggested that yoga may reduce the immune system's proclivity for attacking joint components and therefore may benefit individuals suffering from rheumatoid arthritis. Yoga unquestionably increases range of motion, decreases pain, and improves function in this condition.

Sacroiliac Joint Derangement

We're prone to having these two crucial joints below our waists and above our buttocks become misaligned in part because they support the whole weight of the body above the waist. These complex, irregular joints have a tiny range of motion. Any strenuous activity—twisting, pulling, running, lifting—may force one part of these structures beyond its normal range of motion and concentrate weight where it doesn't belong. This may be extremely painful. Usually the pain is along the margins of the joint, but sometimes it is so severe that it spreads to the low back, hip, and/or abdomen and mimics neurological sciatica.

One characteristic of the pain of SI joint derangement is that it gets worse with certain motions, for instance lifting the feet to get into or out of a car, getting out of bed in the morning, bending down with locked knees and reaching up while in a standing position. If you have neurological signs such as numbness or tingling, chances are it isn't due to SI derangement.

Fortunately, if do you have SI derangement, you can work on it over time with many different yoga poses. Three of my favorites for this condition are Floating Tadasana, Marichyasana, and Gomukhasana. Unlike a dislocation in, say, your shoulder joint, it is unusual for the sacroiliac joint to "pop" back into place and pain to cease at that moment. The more usual course is that the bones move little by little over a period of time until the pain completely disappears.

Spinal Stenosis

Tiny nerves and their roots can be squeezed in openings too narrow for them, causing all sorts of neurological consequences from pain and paraesthesias to numbness and weakness.This is spinal stenosis, a neurological condition, like a pinched nerve. There is a difference, however. A pinched nerve is the compression of a nerve root or nerve roots at the point where it exits it the spinal canal and travels out into the body. Spinal stenosis is nerve compression that occurs inside the spinal canal, involving nerves that come down vertically from the brain. In the lumbar spine these are the same nerve fibers or rootlets that form inside the spinal canal at the T11, T12 level and exit the spine at lower levels. If these fibers are compressed after they join together, it's a radiculopathy or "root disorder." If the compression occurs during the fibers' vertical transit from the brain, before they form the root, the condition is known as spinal stenosis. These nerve(s) are squeezed into a small space before they exit the spinal cord, causing pain that is often localized far away in the areas they serve.

Why does this narrowness occur? The problem may be congenital; the space the nerves travel through may just be narrow from birth. However, as people get older, and often by the time an individual reaches the age of sixty-five or seventy-five, everyone's spine gets narrower due to osteoarthritis: The bones get thicker, the spaces that separate them get smaller. This isn't a problem unless the nerves rub against the inside of the spinal canal, become irritated, and swell. That makes them fit even less well and causes more friction. This is the beginning of a vicious cycle.

The spinal nerves in question are thickest when the spine is straight. Like rubber bands, they stretch and get thinner if you arch your back. If you have spinal stenosis, pain is usually worse when you're standing up or lying down—that is, when the spine is straight. When you're sitting the pain is likely to abate, at least somewhat, because your arched back stretches and thins the nerves so that they take up less space inside the bony spinal canal. Other manifestations of spinal stenosis may be numbness, weakness, tingling, and burning, usually located more or less symmetrically in both feet and ankles and the outsides of the calves or thighs. Sometimes there is also loss of bowel and bladder control. A combination of MRI and EMG (electromyography) is a good way to diagnose spinal stenosis. In my opinion, a combination of medications such as steroids and yoga is the first treatment of choice. Unfortunately and fortunately, surgery is frequently necessary and usually quite successful.

Progressive spinal stenosis is best treated surgically, before the point where pain is increasing and ability to withstand surgery is diminishing. Widening the canal is the simplest, safest, and most effective surgical option, but there are a number of cases where it is not indicated or doesn't work. Fusion of vertebrae is now safer and more beneficial than it has ever been throughout its checkered history.

Other Causes of Neurological Pain

In individuals who have osteoarthritis, a condition that often strikes older people, the spinal canal may gradually but progressively narrow the spinal column in diameter. Radiculopathies and stenosis can also result from a trauma like a fall, or from a fracture or a tumor. Physical yoga may be recommended to treat side effects of a tumor. It can be helpful, if done with care, for a fracture. In my opinion yoga can help reduce the likelihood of fractures by counteracting osteoarthritis. I have included a number of poses that may help relieve pain and sciatica from radiculopathies and stenosis, especially if caused by osteoarthritis and herniated disc.

There are other instances where sciatica strikes that have nothing to do with the back. I have been studying piriformis syndrome for more than twenty years. Sciatica is often caused when the piriformis muscle in the buttock presses on the sciatic nerve. The muscle can go into a lengthy spasm, causing a lot of pain at the site and sometimes producing pain that shoots down the leg.

PART II

Poses by Diagnosis

CHAPTER 6

Musculoskeletal Pain

Pain that is not due to anatomical abnormalities is usually musculoskeletal. It may go away by itself. It usually responds to gentle treatment like yoga. A wrench, a sprain, a strain, poor posture, or emotional stress may produce pain in the lower back. Overworked, tired muscles may go into spasm. To make matters worse, adaptation to that discomfort can cause pain to arise in the upper back and cervical regions.

Muscle spasm is an intense, prolonged, and involuntary contraction. The pain it causes is often grossly underestimated by otherwise excellent clinicians, partially because it does not show up on imaging studies and may occur without detectable medical abnormality. However, a good physician can usually treat spasm without any special equipment.

In a way, spasm stems from an engineering imperfection that occurs in all muscles. Capillaries, which supply fuel and the oxygen to burn it and carry away the waste products of this metabolism, are actually narrowed significantly during muscle contraction. This happens exactly when the muscles are working and these functions are

needed most. As a consequence, one of the by-products of metabolism, lactic acid, builds up in the immediate vicinity of the muscle
fibers. The lactic acid and other irritants cause further contraction of
the muscle fibers, making the condition even worse, and even less
under direct voluntary control.

Yoga poses for musculoskeletal pain concentrate on relieving
this vicious cycle by stretching to elongate muscle fibers mechani-
cally and by means of reflexes. Just the act of increasing the distance
the muscle spans will stretch it and thereby open the capillaries and
ameliorate the condition and its causes. Reflexes initiated by the
stretch itself and by the activation of antagonist muscles will sub-
stantially reduce the tendency for spasm to recur. I have discussed
this in the first chapter.

There is a reason I recommend starting by holding yoga poses
for ten to fifteen seconds, gradually increasing to thirty seconds, and
then to one to two minutes or longer, and that is related to relieving
pain. Stretched for that period of time, muscles will relax and tend to
stay that way. If you stretch too quickly, too violently, or for too
short a time, the muscles will snap back like rubber bands, and the
pain will remain or recur. The first pose in this chapter works differently; holding it for much longer periods of time is desirable.

1. VIPARITA KARANI
Inverted Lake

BENEFITS: Bridges the gap between forward bends and inverted
(upside-down) poses, and has some of the advantages of both:
Stretches hamstrings, drains blood from lower extremities. Good for
headache; produces calm. Good for back pain during pregnancy.

WARNING: Take care to do this pose with minimal elevation if you
have glaucoma, congestive heart failure, or pulmonary congestion.

Three modified variations for beginners:
VIPARITA KARANI MODIFIED (VERSION 1) Lie on the floor
with the backs of the calves and ankles resting on a chair or couch
or close to a wall. Straighten knees, extend arms overhead, palms

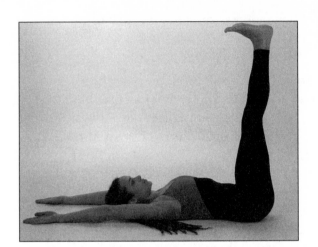
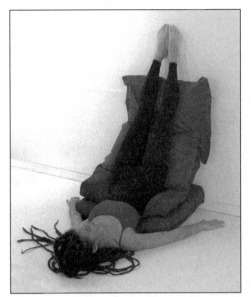

upward. Shoulder blades should be flat and close together. Relax your neck and face. Palms face upward. Stay in this pose for one to three minutes.

After that time, bend one knee, bringing that leg to the floor. Then repeat with the other leg.

VIPARITA KARANI MODIFIED (VERSION 2) Sit on a cushion. Bring the left leg up onto pillows placed on a chair or couch or against the wall. Lie down as you bring the other leg up into a parallel position. Now straighten your knees and let gravity push your shoulder blades down toward your lower back. Bring the shoulder blades together, opening the chest. Relax your abdominal, chest, and neck muscles. Try to relax all the muscles of the head and face. Put hands on your abdomen, at your sides pointing toward your feet, or overhead and pointing backward. Breathe evenly for ten to fifteen minutes.

You will be very relaxed when you come out of the pose and there is little danger, but do it carefully. Raise one leg up so that the calf is no longer on the seat of the chair or couch. Pressing down with your hands slightly, bring one foot to the floor. Ease yourself over to the side so you can bring your other leg down. Alternatively, if it's a small chair, bring the one leg down to the left and then bring the right leg down to the right.

VIPARITA KARANI MODIFIED (VERSION 3) Use more cushions and pillows. Position yourself as you did in the previous pose, but higher, so the feet are extended and parallel. Arms rest on pillows. Close your eyes. Breathe slowly and smoothly for ten to fifteen minutes, going from head to toe, trying to relax each muscle in your body. Skip over nothing.

To get out of this pose, carefully take your left leg off of the chair or couch and place as much of the sole of the left foot as possible on the floor. "Walk" the leg farther away from the pillows until there is room to bring down the right leg. Wait a short time, then roll from your back to your side.

2. JANUSIRSASANA
Head to the Knee (forward bend)

BENEFITS: Increases flexibility, reduces spasm in hamstrings and adductors.

WARNING: Bending too intensely may strain or even sprain hamstrings.

JANUSIRSASANA MODIFIED Sit squarely on the floor, extending the left leg so that the foot is firmly vertical and the toes point toward the ceiling. Bend the right knee, placing the sole of the right foot high up against the inner left thigh so that it and the right shin form a ninety-degree angle. Place palms on the floor, fingers pointing forward. Keep the back and the left knee straight. Press down and backward on the floor with your hands and fingers, inclining your torso toward the left foot. The most important things are to keep the extended knee fully extended and to keep

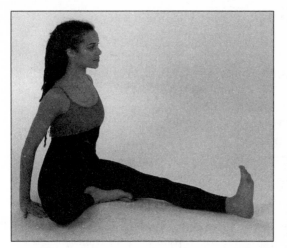 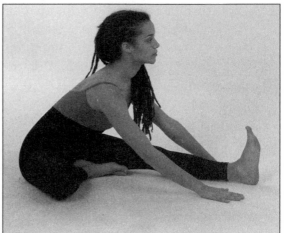

the back straight. Like all yoga poses, holding a moderate stretch for a longer time is preferable to a more intense, shorter version. Breathe slowly for ten to fifteen seconds, then release the pressure from your hands, come up to vertical, and reverse the pose, stretching the other leg.

JANUSIRSASANA REGULAR Sit squarely on the floor, extending the left leg so that the foot is firmly vertical and the toes point toward the ceiling. Bend the right knee, placing the sole of the right foot high up against the inner left thigh so that it and the right shin form a ninety-degree angle. Keeping your back straight, inhale and bend evenly from the hips—not from the lumbar or thoracic spine— toward the foot. Do not bend your neck, but keep facing straight forward, not down. Exhale as you descend. As you come forward, align your sternum with the inside of the extended leg. Since you are doing this pose with the left leg extended, grasp your right wrist with your left hand, beyond the left foot. Relax the muscles of your back and chest and arms. Then work to relax the back thigh muscles of your extended leg. One way to do this is to contract the quadriceps muscle, which extends the left knee. This activates a reflex that relaxes the hamstrings. Stay in the position for fifteen seconds at first, but gradually work up to one minute on each side. Unless otherwise noted, this goes for all the following poses.

To come out of this pose, release your hands. Keeping your back straight, slowly draw your entire spine back until you're sitting with your back in a vertical position.

3. PASCHIMOTTANASANA
West Posture
(Yoga is traditionally done facing east; since this pose stretches
the back of the body, it's named for the west.)

BENEFITS: Increases hamstring, gluteal, and lumbar flexibility; reduces spasm; calms the practitioner; isometrically balances upper and lower extremity muscle tone; lowers blood pressure; and relieves constipation.

CAUTION: May cause gastric problems or discomfort if done on a full stomach.

PROP: Yoga strap.

PASCHIMOTTANASANA MODIFIED Sit squarely and evenly on the floor. Legs are parallel and extended, ankles touching, feet vertical. Slowly move your hands down your legs. Use your hands for balance and support. Keep your back straight and gradually move your torso forward toward your extended feet. Continue to keep your back straight as you walk your hands forward as close to your feet as possible. You can loop a strap around your feet to bring yourself forward rather than down. Resist letting your legs turn outward or bending your knees, even if it means a less intense forward bend. Keeping your back straight, grasp your calves, ankles, or feet at the lowest point you can reach. Relax everything but the hands. Breathe evenly. Start by holding the pose for fifteen seconds, then half a minute, and continue until you are holding it for as long as five minutes. There should be some discomfort from the stretch, but it should not be extreme.

Leave this pose by releasing your hands. Come up slowly, keeping your back straight. Use your hands on your legs for support as your torso rises to vertical.

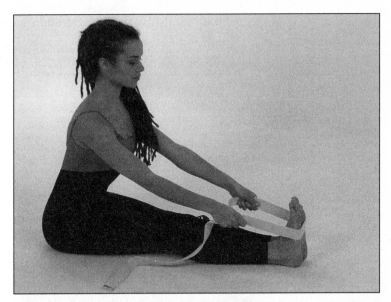

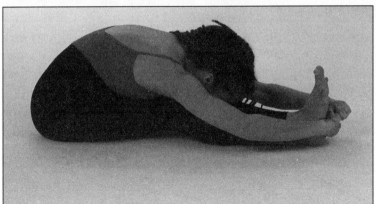

PASCHIMOTTANASANA REGULAR Sit squarely on the floor with both legs extended, knees straight, feet vertical, ankles touching. Inhale, open chest, pull in stomach. Keeping back straight, exhale while bending forward from the waist or hips as far as possible. Reach as far forward as possible, until you can grasp your right wrist with your left hand, beyond the foot, and the backs of both hands face the soles of your feet. Bring head forward, not down. Bring navel toward thighs. Breathe slowly, pausing between breaths. Start at ten to fifteen seconds, continue extending the pose gradually to as long as half an hour.

To exit this pose, release your hands. Inhale as you slowly come up to a sitting position.

4. PARSVOTTANASANA
Stretching of the Flank

BENEFITS: Improves posture, reducing pain between shoulder blades. Stretching the entire back of the body and legs, one side at a time, it relieves muscle spasm and improves flexibility.

CAUTION: Do not do this pose if you are pregnant. You need to digest for four to five hours after eating before doing this pose.

PARSVOTTANASANA MODIFIED Stand with legs three feet apart. Turn the left foot out ninety degrees, and the right foot in thirty degrees. With arms behind the back, interlace fingers with upward-facing palms. Take a half turn to the left (ninety degrees) so that your navel is pointing in the same direction as the left foot. Push hands down toward the floor, straightening the elbows and bringing the shoulders back, down, and together. Keeping knees and spine straight, gently throw your head back and inhale. Then exhale and bring the entire torso forward toward the left leg and thigh. Bend only at the hips. Feel the stretch in the left hamstring and the back of the left calf. Shoulder blades should continue to move toward each other and down. Keep fingers interlaced. Bring your hands farther down toward your buttocks again. Stay in the pose for fifteen seconds on each side, breathing slowly through the nostrils. Gradually increase the time to one minute. To change sides, first bring the torso to vertical, then turn it and feet back to the initial forward position. Then turn the right foot out ninety degrees and the left foot in thirty degrees. Turn your torso so that your navel is facing in the same direction as the right foot. Then exhale. Continue on the right as you did on the left.

To exit this pose, bring your torso up to vertical and release your hands to relax your arms. If you choose, you can place your hands

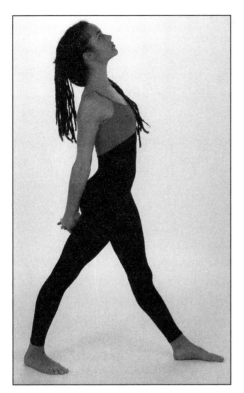 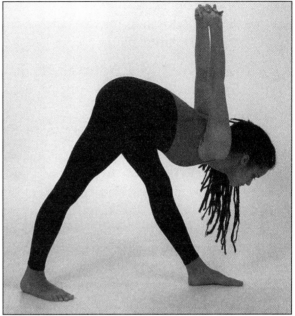

on your thigh for support as you raise your torso to vertical. Bring your hands to your sides. Turn your hips and feet to straight-ahead position. As you inhale, bring your feet together.

PARSVOTTANASANA REGULAR Proceed as above, until you exhale and bring the entire torso forward toward the right leg and thigh. Keeping the head elevated and neck extended (curved back), bring the navel close to the right thigh. Now raise your straightened arms up and away from your back, toward the top of the extended head. Pull the shoulder blades back and down toward the buttocks again. Proceed to completion as in the modified version just above. At first hold this pose for ten to fifteen seconds. Gradually increase to one minute on each side.

To leave the pose, lower your arms as you raise your torso to vertical. When your hands rest against the lumbar spine, release them. Turn feet and torso forward.

5. SUPTA VIRASANA
Lying-Down Hero

BENEFITS: Relaxation; relieves stiffness by stretching hip joint flexors and abdominal muscles; helps correct sacroiliac joint derangement, alleviating pain.

WARNING: If you are pregnant, do this pose cautiously, possibly using a cushion for back support. Beginners must sit on a cushion to avoid knee injury.

PROP: Two blankets.

SUPTA VIRASANA MODIFIED Sit on haunches with pillow or blanket between shins, and knees as close together as possible. Feet are parallel behind you, soles facing upward and heels far enough apart so buttocks fit between them. Straighten back from lumbar spine to the nape of the neck. Place the backs of your hands on the tops of the knees for a few moments. Then lean back until you can place your hands, one at a time, on the floor behind you. Fingers point toward the toes. Breathe evenly and quietly with your mouth closed for ten to fifteen seconds.

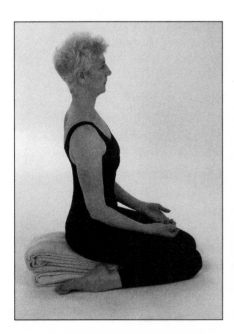
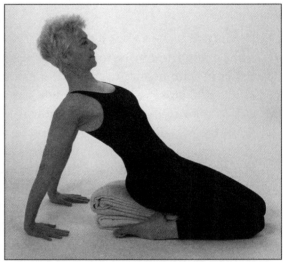

To leave the pose, straighten up to the kneeling position. Then lean forward on all fours.

SUPTA VIRASANA REGULAR Sit on your haunches with your knees together. Your shins are spread enough so your buttocks can fit beneath the heels. Sit squarely on your "sit" (ischial) bones. Balance for a moment with backs of hands on knees. Then lean back until you can place your hands, one at a time, on the floor behind you. Fingers point toward the toes. Then bend the elbows until your entire forearms are resting on the floor. Slide the arms forward until your shoulders, upper, and finally midback are all resting on the floor. At last, bring your arms straight over your head, so that the backs of the arms and hands are resting on the floor, fingers pointing in the same direction as the toes. Hold this pose for ten to fifteen seconds, stretching out the back and the backs of the hands and arms.

To exit, bring your arms back to your sides, palms up. Put weight on your elbows as you bend them, pressing symmetrically and hard enough, to raise your torso to the seated position. Gradually straighten your elbows as you rise. Breathe in as you come out of the pose.

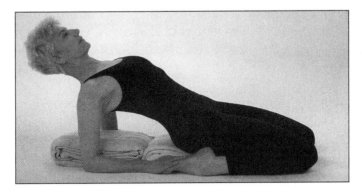

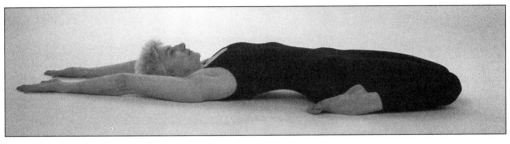

6. MARICHYASANA I
Sage Marishi—Grandfather of the Sun God

BENEFITS: Good for back pain due to muscle spasm because it provides a stretch for the back of the body from the heels to the nape of the neck. Improves hip extensor, abductor, and adductor range, as well as therapeutically opening the sacroiliac joint and thoracic spine. All this helps one adapt to lower back problems and avoid future lower back pain. Excellent for upper-lower extremity coordination and weight control.

WARNING: Do not do this pose if you are pregnant. If you have problems with knee joints, you should flex the knees less. Don't do this pose for four to five hours after eating.

PROP: Small pillow or blanket.

MARICHYASANA I MODIFIED Sit on the floor, left leg extended. Bend the right knee until the knee is directly over the foot: i.e., the shin is vertical. The right foot is parallel to the left thigh, and flush with it. Keeping your torso vertical, place both hands on the floor, fingers facing forward. Gently but firmly press your hands and fingers downward and backward, using your abdominal muscles to move the torso directly forward as much as possible. Keep your back

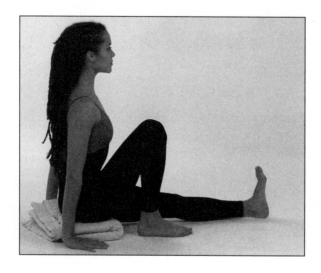

straight; the idea is to bend at the hips and the lowest part of your back, nowhere else. Breathe evenly, attempting to inflate both lungs equally. Stay in the pose for fifteen to thirty seconds.

To get out of this pose, gently release your palms and relax your abdominal muscles. Straighten the right knee. Change legs.

MARICHYASANA I REGULAR Sit on the floor, left leg extended, left foot firm and vertical. Bend the right knee until the knee is directly over the foot and the shin is vertical. The foot of the bent leg is parallel to the left thigh and flush with it. Lean forward without bending to the right or left. Curl the right arm around the right shin just below the knee. Grasp the left foot with the left hand. Maintaining a straight back, push backward with the right upper arm and pull forward with the left hand. Lower your navel to the inner left thigh. Don't worry about how low your head is going. Keep both shoulders level in the forward and vertical directions. Flex your left quadriceps to relax the left hamstring. Tighten your abdominal muscles to relax your lower back muscles. When you have stretched your hamstrings and lower back sufficiently, remain in the pose for ten to fifteen seconds, breathing evenly and calmly.

To exit the pose, release the left hand and bring the right arm forward, allowing your torso to rise again to vertical. Then repeat the pose by straightening the right leg and bringing the left shin to vertical.

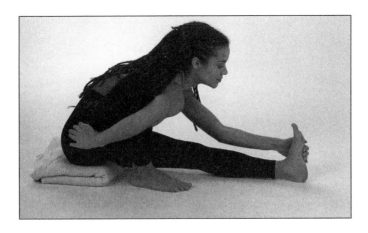

There are some poses that are described and pictured elsewhere in the book for other diagnoses that may also be helpful for musculoskeletal complaints. These poses are in order from acute to chronic pain:

SUPTA PADANAGUSTHASANA—Holding Big Toe While Supine

UPAVISTHA KONASANA—Seated Angle

UTTHITA PARSVAKONASANA—Side at an Angle Pose

HALASANA—Plow

CHAPTER 7

Herniated Nucleus Pulposis

(Herniated Disc,
Pinched Nerve Root)

In everyday parlance, "pinched nerve" roughly describes what physicians call herniated nucleus pulposis, or herniated disc. That's only an approximation of the truth. A herniated nucleus pulposis and a herniated disc are the same thing, but a pinched nerve is something else.

If the disc between L4 and L5 should break open at its back edge, where such ruptures almost invariably occur, first its contents will leak out and press backward into the small openings through which the nerve roots pass as they leave the spinal cord. This initial event is what takes place when a disc is herniated. As a result, partly because it is occupied by the substance that was inside the disc, the space inside the spinal cord decreases. Then, the space decreases further, partly because the L4 vertebra lowers, reducing the size of the space. Third, an inflammatory reaction brings fluids, white cells, and reactant biochemical agents to the region, adding to the congestion and inflammation in the area. These three factors—disc material pressing on nerve openings, decreased space, and increased inflammation of the nerve and its linings—are what cause the "pinched nerve." Of course there are also other causes of pinched nerve, such as degenerative joint disease, swelling of the ligaments, foreign objects, fractures, abscesses, and, rarely, tumors.

When one has a herniated disc or pinched nerve, there is often accompanying sciatica. There may be numbness, tingling, or electric shocks with burning hot or cold sensations. You may have weakness that prevents you from walking on your heels. Just going to bed might seem like the thing to do, though getting up is extremely laborious and painful. Some feel as though a leg is suddenly heavier or "not part of me" somehow. Of course when one feels this way, the rational and proper thing to do is see a physician. Then the MRI or EMG will help make the diagnosis.

Ironically, although a herniated disc is permanent and never repairs itself structurally, it may not hurt at the moment it ruptures or even later. In 1991, Dr. Maureen Jensen canvassed one hundred people with no history of low back pain and found that at least thirty had significant disc abnormalities.[1] An individual can have a herniated disc and back pain that is unrelated, and actually caused by something else.

I use the six-week rule when helping a patient decide on treatment options. If he or she has a herniated disc and extreme pain that is not relieved by conservative means after four to six weeks, I have found that surgery can be very effective. Studies have shown, however, that the pain of herniated disc usually abates over time (which could be years), whether or not the patient has surgery. If you don't have surgery will you always be weak? That's a question of whether the herniated disc and its consequences actually sever any nerve fibers. If those fibers are severed, there may be lasting weakness or numbness.

That brings us to the other reason for surgery: There are danger signals. If you have adverse changes such as numbness that ascends from your feet toward your knees or hips, increasing weakness, or are losing bowel or bladder control, then this is no time for yoga. Put the book down and make your way quickly and carefully to medical attention. This problem is rare. I have found that usually medication and physical therapy, coupled with a judicious program you can do at home, will take you out of pain.

When determining what kind of exercise is appropriate and which yoga exercises may be of most benefit, it is important to me to distinguish between a newly herniated disc and one that ruptured some time ago. A disc that herniated last week and caused sudden, unremitting pain is different from the disc that ruptured eight months ago and that still bothers you chronically but not to the degree it did when the injury first occurred. In my opinion there is a dramatic gradation from the mild movements appropriate for someone who is in great pain from a recent injury and the somewhat more strenuous activities most useful to the individual who is trying to keep in shape to control pain and prevent flare-ups.

In what follows, as in all the other chapters, the earlier poses are for more acute pain, and later ones are more appropriate for chronic conditions. Do not go whole hog into them. Be tentative and experimental. Your curiosity about your body and how you can help yourself out of pain may very well restore you to greater health.

1. STANDING KAPOTASANA
Pigeon

BENEFITS: Elongates and therefore thins spinal cord and nerve roots while moving disc material out of their path. Increases range of motion of entire spine. Relieves fatigue in lower back.

WARNING: Do not do this pose if you are pregnant. If doing this pose produces dizziness, arch less intensely and come out of the pose more slowly.

STANDING KAPOTASANA MODIFIED Stand with feet parallel and a solid wall about eighteen inches behind you. Your hands are at your sides. Bring your hips slightly forward and at the same time put your forearms above your head and lean back until your palms are flat against the wall. Fingers point backward and down. Lean backward and breathe slowly for ten to fifteen seconds. To exit, raise your head and hands, then lower your hands to your sides.

STANDING KAPOTASANA REGULAR Lean backward as in the modified version of the pose, but keep going until your fingertips touch the wall. Use fingertips to crawl downward as much as you are able. Emphasize arching the chest, not the lumbar spine. Do not

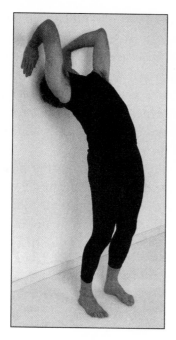 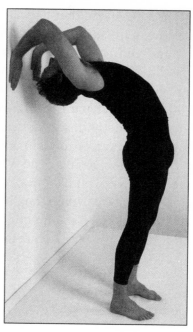

strain. Breathe in your chest, not in your stomach, for ten to fifteen seconds. Then gradually crawl up the wall. Slowly push away from the wall. Your chest stays in a forward position. Bring throat forward, then chin, then head.

2. BHUJANGASANA
Cobra

BENEFITS: Pulls disc material away from nerve rootlets by stretching the front of the neck, chest, abdomen, and thighs. Reduces pain. Helps open lumbosacral, thoracic, and hip joints.

WARNING: Do not do this pose if you are more than three months pregnant.

BHUJANGASANA MODIFIED Lie on stomach facedown. Your elbows are about at nipple level. Palms are flat on the floor, fingers spread. Without pressing hands down, lift forehead, eyebrows, nose, chin, and throat off the floor. Hold for ten to fifteen seconds.

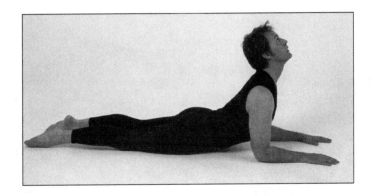

BHUJANGASANA REGULAR When you have gone as far as you are able at the end of the modified version of this pose, apply slight pressure to your hands. Keeping navel on the floor, lift your head and press it back. It's impossible, but look back over your head as if you were trying to see your heels.

To get out of both the modified and regular versions of this pose, simultaneously release your head and lower your abdomen. Any weight on your hands and arms will decrease. Place your right arm so that it will cushion your forehead as your head lowers to the floor. Then push with your left arm to turn over.

3. USTRASANA
Camel

BENEFITS: Increases room for nerves exiting spine. This pose is also helpful for spinal stenosis.

WARNING: This is generally a very safe pose, but do it cautiously if you are pregnant.

USTRASANA MODIFIED Sit on heels with knees together. Grasp heels. Straighten your elbows as you lift the pubic bone and press it forward, resting more weight at the point of contact between the heels of your hands and the heels of your feet. Hold for ten to fifteen seconds.

USTRASANA REGULAR Continue pressing pelvis forward and up. Slowly move your head backward, lift sternum and solar plexus

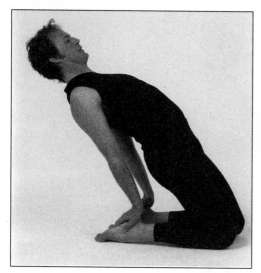 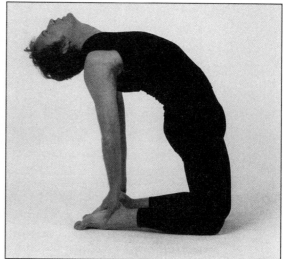

toward the ceiling. This diminishes the weight on hands and arms.

As you exhale to come out of the pose, reduce the pressure on your abdomen and pubic bones so that you are sitting down again. Your center of gravity will now be more or less under your feet. Bring your hands to your lap. Place your right palm on the floor beside your right thigh. Use it to support you as you release your left leg. Alternatively, come forward on all fours.

4. UTKATASANA
Powerful, Fierce

BENEFITS: Strengthens lower back support muscles, protecting the nerves. Coordinates the back and leg muscles to reduce postural pressure on nerves.

WARNING: Do not do this pose if you are pregnant. People with balance problems should do this against a wall. People with hypertension should moderate the intensity and duration of this pose.

NOTE: There are three differences between the modified and regular poses. First, there is less knee flexion in the modified version. Second, the modified version is done with your back near or against a wall. Third, heels remain on the floor in the regular version.

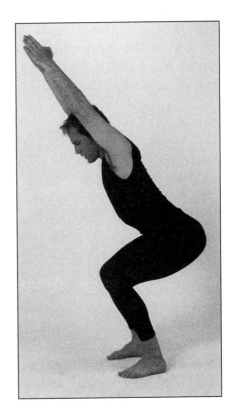

UTKATASANA MODIFIED AND REGULAR Stand with feet parallel, directly under hips. Bring arms over head. Hands are together, thumbs holding palms flush with each other. Slowly bend knees, keeping back stretched as straight and heels as close to the floor as possible. Descend as far as possible. Hold for ten to fifteen seconds, breathing evenly with mouth closed.

The normal way to exit this pose is to straighten your knees and then release your thumbs. Bring your arms down as your exhale. However, if you feel that you are losing your balance or tiring, first lower your hands and then straighten your knees.

5. TRIKONASANA
Triangle

BENEFITS: Stretches and thins Ligamentum Flavum (a ligament just behind the nerves inside the spinal column, down the entire length of the spine). Relieves sciatica-causing pressure on spinal nerves.

WARNING: Overdoing this pose can sprain hamstrings and adductor muscles on inside of thighs.

TRIKONASANA MODIFIED Stand with feet three feet apart. Turn left foot out ninety degrees and right foot in thirty degrees. Stretch arms and fingertips out horizontally as far as possible at shoulder height. Inhale and then breathe evenly for ten to fifteen seconds.

Turn feet so that they are facing forward to exit the pose. As you exhale, bring your arms down to your sides.

TRIKONASANA REGULAR The modified pose is the first part of the regular pose. To do the regular pose, just continue in the modified version to stretch your arms out horizontally, palms down. Then, moving the torso all at once without curving the spine, lower the left hand to the left foot or shin. Right arm becomes vertical, remaining in a direct line with the left arm. Keeping the right foot on the floor, turn the right knee outward. but don't move the left leg. This lengthens the right groin and widens the left groin. Keep right ribs low; they should not bulge upward. Your torso should be horizontal, the extended arms vertical—your whole body in the same plane. As a guide, you should be able to see your right thumb with your left eye. Breathe symmetrically for ten to fifteen seconds at first, moving in small increments toward one minute on each side.

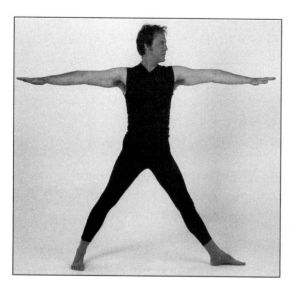
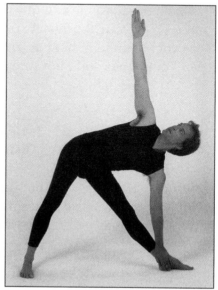

To come out of the pose, bring your torso back to vertical as you inhale, keeping your arms horizontal. Turn your feet so they are facing forward. Relax your arms. Bring your feet together. Repeat the pose on the opposite side.

6. UTTHITA PARSVAKONASANA
Side at an Angle Pose

BENEFITS: Greatly increases balance and coordination. Combats muscle spasm one side at a time. May clear space for nerves exiting the spinal cord.

WARNING: If you have poor balance, do this against a wall.

PROP: A block.

UTTHITA PARSVAKONASANA MODIFIED Stand with your feet five feet apart. Turn the left foot out ninety degrees and the right foot in thirty degrees. Take a breath. As you exhale, bend your left knee ninety degrees, keeping your right leg straight. Place right hand on left thigh. Hold for ten to fifteen seconds.

To exit the pose, straighten your left knee so that you are standing with feet five feet apart. Turn your feet so they are facing forward. Bring your arms to your sides.

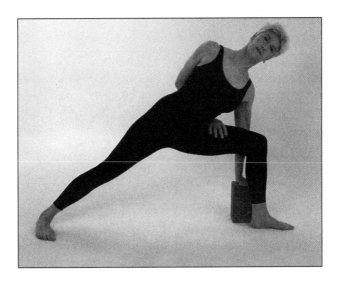

UTTHITA PARSVAKONASANA REGULAR Stand with feet five feet apart. Turn left foot out ninety degrees and right foot in thirty degrees. Take a breath in. As you exhale, bend your left knee ninety degrees keeping your right leg straight. Place your left palm on the floor next to your left foot on the little toe side, and parallel to it. Balance the weight evenly among the left hand, the left foot, and the right foot. Extend the right arm behind the ear, diagonally, palm down. Press the left biceps into the outside of the left knee and the knee outward into the biceps. Revolve the right torso upward, opening the left groin. Then extend the right hand, arm, shoulder, flank, hip, and leg down to the little toe, making the right side of your body a straight line. Breathe smoothly and symmetrically and deeply for ten to fifteen seconds, trying to inflate both lungs equally in spite of the asymmetry of the torso. As you breathe, stretch your right side while supporting and turning it with the left. Do not lean forward or back.

To exit the pose, relax the pressure between biceps and outside of knee. Bring torso to vertical and raise your arms to horizontal as they were when you entered the pose. If this becomes difficult, then keeping the torso vertical, you can press your left hand against your left thigh to straighten the leg, balancing your right hand on the right hip. Then you can remain in this pose, with your shoulder blades down, back, and together, breathing evenly, looking ahead for ten to fifteen seconds.

To continue exiting the pose, turn the feet to a forward and parallel position. Repeat the pose on the opposite side.

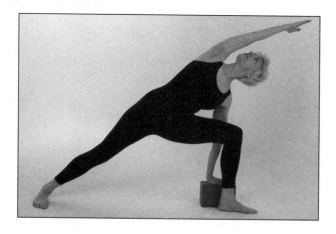

7 . Uttanasana
Intense Stretch

BENEFITS: Opens spaces between vertebrae, may relieve disc pressure. Good for chronic disc problems.

WARNING: Dangerous if you have a newly herniated disc. But if spasm dominates or you have chronic pain from a herniated disc, this is a useful pose. If you are pregnant, do this pose with your palms against a wall in front of you.

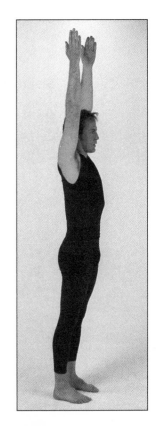

UTTANASANA MODIFIED Stand with feet parallel and directly below hips. Distribute your weight evenly between and within your feet. Make your body and breathing as quiet as possible for twenty seconds. This is a pose in itself and is called Tadasana, Mountain Pose (see 4 in chapter 14, "After Back Surgery," page 183) Breathe in and raise your arms directly over your head. Palms face each other. Arms and legs are in direct line. Stretch your arms up, your legs down as you breathe calmly for ten to fifteen seconds. Retain the even distribution of weight.

To come out of this pose, bring your palms down as you exhale.

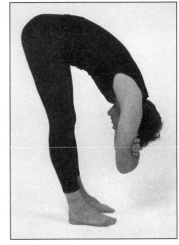

UTTANASANA REGULAR Begin at the end of the modified pose with arms stretched up and legs extended downward. As you exhale, bend slowly but crisply from the hips. Maintaining stretch of torso and legs, place palms on the floor. If you can't get down that far, fold your arms and let gravity pull them (and the rest of your upper body) down as much as possible. Hold the pose for ten to fifteen seconds.

To release: Keep your arms in close to your torso as you come up. If you experience apprehension, then "walk" up your thighs with your hands and fingers, giving your trunk support as you do.

There are some poses that are described and pictured elsewhere in the book for other diagnoses that may also be helpful for herniated nucleus pulposis. They are, in order from acute to chronic pain:

SAVASANA—Corpse Pose

SETU BANDHA SARVANGASANA—Bridge Pose

ADHO MUKHA SVANASANA—Downward-Facing Dog

SUPTA PADANAGUSTHASANA—Holding Big Toe While Supine

CHAPTER 8

Arthritis

Arthritis is an insidiously progressive condition, regardless of its type, of which there are many. The most common include:

- Osteoarthritis, also called degenerative joint disease, affects as many as 32.9 million Americans over the age of forty, according to the National Center for Health Statistics.[1] While it is often considered a "wear-and-tear" condition, there is evidence that nutrition, activity level, gender, and other factors are also significant. Osteoarthritis usually affects fingers and weight-bearing joints, especially the knees, hips, feet, and back.
- Fibromyalgia is classified by the Arthritis Foundation as an arthritis-related condition,[2] which is more common among women than men. It affects fascia, muscles, and their attachments to bones. Symptoms range from pain and stiffness to difficulty sleeping and emotional distress.
- Rheumatoid arthritis is an immune system problem also more common in women than in men. It damages joint linings, cartilage, and bone, causing destructive inflammation and resulting in deformities.

The pain of arthritis may be acute pain that can develop one day and hurt a great deal, or it can be chronic pain that is there most, or all, of the time in varying intensity. In an episode of acute pain, medications and physical therapy can help, and yoga may also bring relief. The key to this, of course, is that by its very nature, an episode of acute pain ends. The chronic pain is harder to deal with, both psychologically and physically. Yoga, slow and steady, is well suited to helping an individual cope with chronic complaints.

Whether pain is chronic or acute, it comes from three sources. First, if a joint is degenerating, you can expect it to hurt. Second, when a degenerating joint is causing discomfort, an individual is less likely to move it; when it does move there is pain in the joint from the stretch of the tightened ligaments, tendons, and joint capsule itself. Last, when a joint is damaged and moves poorly, problems may arise in the ligaments, tendons, and capsules of other joints nearby. For example, if you can't bend your back enough to tie your shoelaces, you may start to use your hip joint more than you did before you had the back problem. Actually, in this situation you're in a double bind because the arthritis in the spine is making it necessary to move the hip more, but the arthritis may also be restricting the hip's range of motion even below its previous levels.

Every joint is the interface of two bones. The collagen that makes up the joint surfaces is secreted by live cells. In the hip bones there are beautifully regular alignments of cells in spheres underneath the joint surface that secrete the collagen. As you get older, the underlying rows of cells and the collagen they secrete come in a bit unevenly on both surfaces. This is exacerbated by normal wear and tear, and when the outside forces on the joint are uneven. When this begins happening to the collagen, it becomes irregular, and instead of being evenly distributed throughout the joint, the pressure in certain spots inside the joint goes up a great deal. At that point, the disruption in the underlying tissue makes those beautifully aligned rows of cells get out of line and begin to produce collagen that has bumps, lumps, and ridges in it. Of course that concentrates the already immense pressure on both joint surfaces, causing more damage.

Yoga works by stretching the joints, ligaments, tendons, and capsules so they don't get as tight as they would otherwise. This

URDHVA MUKHA SVANASANA REGULAR Lie on your stomach, feet a foot apart. Your hands should be beneath your shoulders, palms on the floor, fingers pointing forward. Toes are flexed, i.e., curled away from the floor. Do not bend your hips or knees. Lift your head, brow, bridge of nose, then chin, top of throat, chest, and abdomen until elbows are straight. At this point only palms and tops of feet are on the floor. Breathe, inflating lungs completely, for ten to fifteen seconds.

To get out of the pose, gradually lower your chest from the point just above the navel, where it has left the floor. Unfold your chest, neck, and head, slowly bring your chest, shoulders, and head back to the floor.

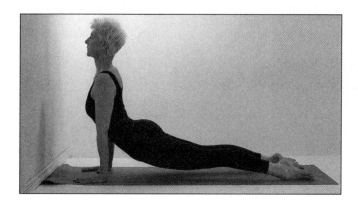

2. ADHO MUKHA SVANASANA
Downward-Facing Dog

BENEFITS: Stretches hip joint and hamstrings, strengthens extensor muscles in spine. Increases upper back, shoulder, and neck mobility

CAUTION: Do the modified pose if you have severe arthritis or rotator cuff problems.

PROP: Mat, optional.

ADHO MUKHA SVANASANA MODIFIED This is the same pose as the modified version of Urdhva Mukha Svanasana (1, above). Stand facing a wall. You should be about eighteen inches away, with your feet directly beneath the hips. Distribute the weight evenly on the feet. Look straight ahead.

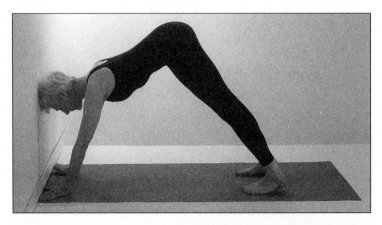

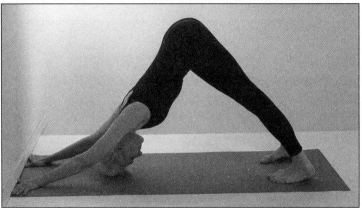

Place your hands high on the wall, well above eye level, a few inches more than shoulder width apart, fingers pointing up. Keeping knees straight, pull your hips back. Bring armpits as close to the wall as possible. The curve of your back will automatically bring your forehead toward the wall. Don't tilt your head. This is an invigorating pose. Breathe slowly and deeply for ten to fifteen seconds.

To exit, push gently against the wall so that your armpits come farther away from the wall. Coordinate this with pulling your hips in toward the wall until you are back in the position from which you started. Lower your hands.

ADHO MUKHA SVANASANA REGULAR Go down on all fours in front of a wall. Place index fingers and thumbs at the base of the wall. Straighten your elbows and knees. Bring your hips up as high as possible and stretch your heels to the floor. Bring your shoulder blades together and back so that your entire back is arched, with your head a continuation of your spine. There should be a ski-slope type of arch from the nape of your neck to your pelvis. You may need to adjust your position by walking your feet forward or back a few inches. Raise your hips up as if someone were pulling you back by holding your belt from behind. Keep your heels on the floor. Breathe quietly for fifteen to twenty seconds.

To come out of the pose, gradually release the pressure on your arms by bending your elbows. Bring your right knee to the floor, then your left knee so that you are on all fours with your head facing the wall.

3. PARIGHASANA
Gate
(looks like a farm gate with a crosspiece)

BENEFITS: Increases spinal range of motion in the side-to-side dimension. Takes stress off the spine by increasing hip range of motion.

WARNING: Do not do this pose if you are pregnant. If balance is severely impaired, this pose can be done facing a wall.

PROP: Mat, optional.

PARIGHASANA BASIS FOR MODIFIED AND REGULAR

NOTE: This is the basis for the modified and regular poses: Kneel with the back erect. Place hands on hips. Then extend arms out horizontally from shoulders, palms down.

PARIGHASANA MODIFIED Extend left leg out to the side. Place left palm on the left knee. Extend right arm over ear, fingers pointing in the same direction as the extended leg. Bend directly to the left side. Do not twist. Breathe as symmetrically as possible for ten to fifteen seconds.

To come out of this pose bring your head back so that your torso and head are vertical and in line. As you do this, slide your left arm

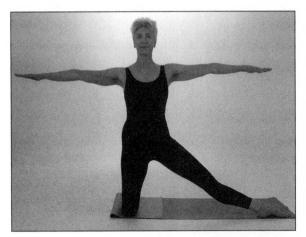

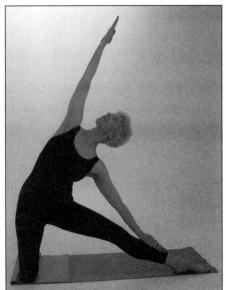

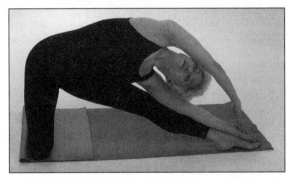

along the top of your extended left leg. Bring the left leg beside the right so that you are kneeling comfortably.

Reverse and do on the other side.

PARIGHASANA REGULAR Continue from the modified pose. Bend further until the right palm meets the left hand on top of the left foot, keeping the left foot on the floor. Arms frame the head at each ear. Breathe calmly for ten to fifteen seconds.

To come out of this pose, release your right (upper) hand and gradually bring it with your head back to the center. Do this while sliding your left arm along the top of your extended left leg until you are kneeling on your right knee with your left leg extended. Bend your left knee and bring the leg to the middle until you are kneeling comfortably.

4. ARDHA PADMA PASCHIMOTTANASANA
Half-Lotus Forward Bend

BENEFITS: Increases flexion of thoracic and lumbar spine. Improves shoulder-blade and upper-arm range of motion, strength, and control. Stretches hamstrings and improves hip range of motion.

WARNING: Do not do the regular version of this pose if you are pregnant. Use extra caution and do not push yourself if you have severe knee arthritis.

PROP: Blanket.

ARDHA PADMA PASCHIMOTTANASANA MODIFIED Sit straight in Dandasana, the Staff Pose (1 in chapter 14, "After Back Surgery," page 179). Take the right leg and place it high on the left thigh so that the foot is close to the groin. Bring the right knee as close to the floor as possible. If your knee doesn't reach the floor you can place a blanket under it. Inhale. Keeping back straight, bend from the hips as much as possible, and press your fingers to the floor. Relax the hamstrings in your left thigh by tightening the quadriceps muscle that extends the knee. Open the chest, attempting to bring the navel toward the left inner thigh. Breathe symmetrically for ten to fifteen seconds, inflating the entire lungs.

To come out of this pose, release the pressure of your fingertips and sit back until your torso is vertical. Release the right foot from its position on the left thigh. You are now in Dandasana. Repeat the pose on the opposite side.

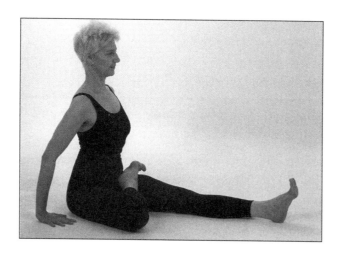

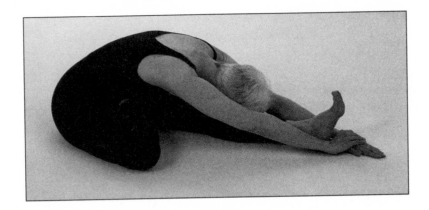

ARDHA PADMA PASCHIMOTTANASANA REGULAR Sit straight in Dandasana. Take the right leg and place it high on the left thigh so that the foot is close to the groin. Bring the right knee as close to the floor as possible. Inhale. Keeping your back straight, bend forward so your abdomen comes in contact with your right foot. Try to relax the muscles in the back of your left thigh by tightening the quadriceps muscle that extends the knee. Stretch the torso and arms forward toward the left foot and beyond its sole. The right hand grasps the left wrist. Let your chin rest on the left leg below the knee. Hold this pose for ten to fifteen seconds, breathing through your nose. Gradually work up to holding it for one minute.

To come out of this pose, release the grasp of the right hand on the left wrist. As you do so both hands slide up the leg and your torso comes to vertical. Release the right foot from its position on the left thigh. You are now in Dandasana. Repeat the pose on the opposite side.

5. PRASARITA PADOTTANASANA
Spread Legs

BENEFITS: Good for lower spine, sacroiliac, and hip joints. Stretches hamstrings and adductors.

WARNING: If your have narrow angle glaucoma, discuss this pose with your ophthalmologist before trying it.

PROP: Stable card-table chair.

PRASARITA PADOTTANASANA MODIFIED Stand with feet parallel and about thirty-six inches apart. Bend forward and place palms on the seat of a chair. Arch your back as much as possible. At first hold for ten to fifteen seconds. Elbows are straight. Head is up and back as far as possible. As time goes on and you practice this pose, use lower and lower supports for your hands, letting the torso descend further.

To come out of this pose, if the chair has arms on it, put your right hand on the arm of the chair. Use pressure on your upper limbs to bring yourself to vertical, bringing left hand to the chair arm as soon as possible. With an armless chair, bend your knees as you raise your torso to vertical. You are now standing, looking at the chair. Bring your legs together.

PRASARITA PADOTTANASANA REGULAR Stand with feet four feet apart and parallel. Then lower your palms until they are flat on the floor; fingertips should be in line with the toes. Arch the entire back and neck, raising your head as much as possible. Breathe quietly for ten to fifteen seconds. Now grasp the outsides of your ankles with your hands. This pose can be extended even farther. To exit, place hands on hips and straighten torso to vertical.

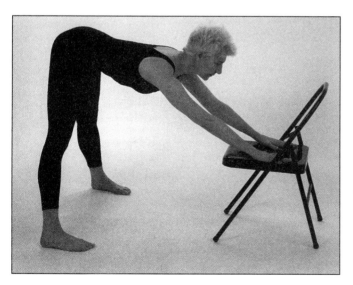
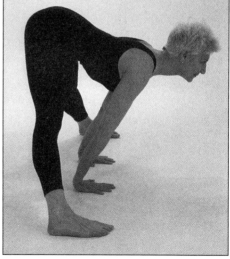

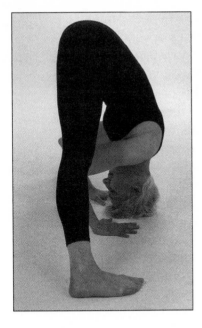

PRASARITA PADOTTANASANA REGULAR (EXTENDED) Keep your back and neck straight. Pull your torso down so your ears are in line with your ankles. Resist the tendency to breathe deeply so as to avoid tightening some of the muscles you're trying to stretch. Breathe quietly for ten to fifteen seconds.

To exit the pose, release your grasp on your ankles. Gradually, with back arched, bring your head and torso first to horizontal, pausing with your hands on the floor, your fingertips in line with your toes. Breathe smoothly for ten to fifteen seconds. Then place hands on hips and return to vertical until you are standing. Bring your legs together.

6. SETU BANDHA SARVANGASANA
Bridge Pose

BENEFITS: Improves strength of the entire back and abdomen. Increases range of motion of these regions and opens the chest.

CAUTION: Do not do this pose if you are pregnant or have glaucoma. If you have high blood pressure, reduce the time that you hold the pose and the angle at which you do it.

PROP: Stable card-table chair.

SETU BANDHA SARVANGASANA MODIFIED Stand facing the chair. Hold the chair back, insert the right foot into the space between the back and the seat of the chair, and as you do so, sit on the chair. Then bend the left knee and insert the left foot beside the right so that both feet are stationed on the floor behind the chair. (NOTE: Use care. If the chair begins to tip, then try sitting a little farther from the chair's back. If it still seems unstable, a partner can help you enter and leave the pose.) Slide farther into the space between the chair back and seat until your buttocks emerge almost fully behind the chair. Hold the chair back with both hands, and

CHAPTER 9

Sacroiliac Joint Derangement

Sacroiliac (SI) joint derangement is one of the most underdiagnosed, undertreated, and exceedingly painful back problems. Many medical professionals have a poor understanding of it, and many otherwise excellent practitioners are downright skeptical of its existence. Those who feel the pain, however, are far from doubtful. It's the sort of sudden, severe pain that provides great incentive to find relief. Thankfully, once you have ruled out other conditions and are convinced this is the problem, there is something you can do about SI joint derangement.

The sacroiliac joints are located on each side of your back, not far below the waist, in line with the inner margins of kidneys. Unlike your knee and ankle joints, which are flat and horizontal and make structural sense because they hold you up and steady, the sacroiliac joints are almost vertical. All the weight in the upper body, all our twisting movements and other types of action must be supported by these vertical joints. Because of their structure and placement, these joints need powerful ligaments to hold them in the proper position. The ligaments typically withstand tremendous forces. Unfortunately,

gradually lean back until your spine is on the seat of the chair. Your shoulder blades should be on, not off, the edge of the seat. Let your neck gradually relax, allowing your head to descend to a comfortable level. Breathe slowly and evenly with mouth closed for ten to fifteen seconds.

To exit the pose, retain the head and neck in their extended position while pulling your torso up with your arms. Then straighten the head and neck. Slide your hips some distance toward the front of the chair, but remain seated. Carefully move your hips to the right and bend your left knee to extricate the left leg and place it on the floor beside the chair. Stand on the left foot while holding on to the back of the chair. Pull your right foot back until you can put it or your right knee on the seat of the chair. After gaining full balance, bring your right foot to the floor and release the chair back.

Setu Bandha Sarvangasana Modified (Intermediate) This is essentially the same as the first version, with a significant difference. After leaning back, with the shoulder blades firmly supported by the edge of the seat of the chair, carefully release your grip on the chair back. Slowly raise both arms to vertical, then lower them behind you, further opening the armpits and chest. The backs of your fingernails may reach to the floor. Let your neck gradually relax while your head descends as far as it can comfortably. Breathe slowly and evenly with mouth closed for ten to fifteen seconds.

To exit the pose, keep your head and neck in their extended position while you slowly return your hands to the lower part of the chair back. Use your elbows to help pull your torso up with your arms. Then straighten the head and neck. Slide your hips a little out of the chair, but remain on it. Carefully move your hips to the right and bend your left knee to extricate the left leg and place it on the floor beside the chair. Stand on the left leg. Still holding on to the back of the chair, pull your right foot back until you can put it or your right knee on the seat of the chair. After gaining full balance, bring your right foot to the floor and release the chair back.

Setu Bandha Sarvangasana Regular Stand facing a folding chair. Hold the chair back, insert the right foot in the space between the back and the seat of the chair, and as you do so, sit on

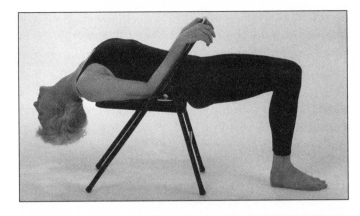

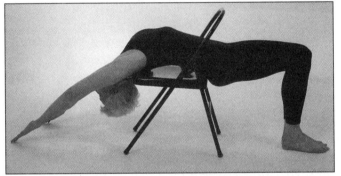

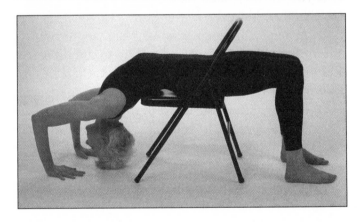

the chair. Then bend the left knee and insert the left foot beside the right so that both feet are firmly on the floor behind the chair. Slide farther into the space between the back and seat until the lower part of each buttock is just slightly behind the chair. Hold the

chair back with both of your hands, and gradually lean back until your spine is on the seat of the chair. As you do, slide your hands down to where the back and seat of the chair meet. Your shoulder blades should be off the edge of the seat. This is how it differs from the modified version.

Let your neck and shoulders and upper chest gradually relax, enabling your head to descend as much as your comfort level allows. Let go of the chair back and bend your elbows ninety degrees as you place your palms on the floor, fingers facing your heels. Balance the weight evenly between your two palms. Breathe slowly and evenly with mouth closed for ten to fifteen seconds.

To exit the pose, keep your head and neck in their extended position while you slowly return your hands to the lower part of the chair back. Slide your torso a safe distance farther into the space between the chair back and seat so that your shoulder blades come closer to the edge of the seat of the chair. Use your elbows to help pull your torso up with your arms. Then straighten the head and neck. Slide your hips partially out of the chair, but remain on it. Carefully move your hips to the right and bend your left knee to extricate the left leg and place it on the floor beside the chair. Stand on the left leg. Still holding on to the back of the chair, pull your right foot back until you can put it or your right knee on the seat of the chair. After regaining full balance, bring your right foot to the floor and release the chair back.

There are some additional poses that are described and pictured elsewhere in the book for other diagnoses that may also be helpful for arthritis. They are, in order of acute to chronic pain:

TRIKONASANA—Triangle Pose

MATSYENDRASANA I—Matsyendra was one of the fathers Hatha yoga

PADMASANA—Lotus

PARIVRTTA JANU SIRSASANA—Twisted Head to Knee Pos

partly because of their shape and placement, and because of their dependency on ligaments, these joints are prone to trouble.

The three-dimensional structure of the SI joint is complex and irregular, and it works like a complicated key in a lock with many notches and tabs that must fit exactly into one another. The normal range of motion of this joint is very small—so small it must be measured in millimeters. Unfortunately, when it is out of alignment it doesn't easily return to its proper position the way a shoulder that has lurched out of place may just slide back where it belongs. Instead, the very ligaments whose strength is a powerful ally in strenuous activities become formidable adversaries, holding the joint in misalignment, concentrating all the forward pressure on tiny areas of the joint, causing great pain. Often the joint must move little by little to become realigned. I have found that yoga is a good way to accomplish and maintain realignment. Theory seems to agree.[1]

How do you know if you have SI derangement? The pain is usually fairly localized. It's right there, a sharp pain on one side or both sides of your back, below your waist about two inches on either side of the midline. The pain usually doesn't radiate at all, and never below the knee, but gives you a twinge when you move or when you go from a sitting to standing position. Exiting the backseat of a car can be extremely unpleasant. There's no weakness, no numbness, no tingling, or other neurological symptom. One hallmark of SI joint pain is that it is usually associated with a specific injury, like stepping into a pothole or overenthusiastically paddling a canoe. If you have one leg that is slightly longer than the other, you may be prone to SI derangement. A long bout of this condition may also cause changes in posture and musculature that can result in a leg-length discrepancy. SI joint derangement often coexists with piriformis syndrome (see chapter 12).

You can do a simple test on yourself for SI joint derangement. Lie down flat on an elevated, hard surface like a table, with one side of your body and one buttock slightly off the edge. Use a wall or other furniture for balance. Let one leg hang down over the edge. If it hurts below the small of your back, you may have this problem.

The pain of SI joint derangement is always in the lower back, but some patients mistakenly think the pain is in their hips. If you do have a derangement of this joint, the more quickly it is diagnosed and treated, the better. A relatively new derangement is easier to deal with than one that has been going on for a long time.

If you think you have SI joint derangement, the yoga poses in this chapter will not make the problem worse. The asanas may help in five distinct ways:

- Reduce tone and spasticity of muscles around the joint so that it is less likely to become fixed in the wrong position and stay there.
- Loosen joints near the SI joint, relieving stress on the SI joint in acute episodes and helping to avoid reaggravation that could lead to chronic derangement.
- Improve posture. Poor posture is a major cause of SI joint derangement.
- Open and allow movement of joint into proper position if it is out of alignment.
- Teach accurate, meaningful, functional body awareness so that you may avoid pushing the joint out of position.

The SI joint can be difficult to realign once it has shifted out of its proper position. There is no sensible surgery that is widely practiced with beneficial results. Chiropractic, osteopathy, and physical therapy use the legs as levers in order to move this recalcitrant joint into the correct position. Yoga is much more than just an alternative method for treating SI joint derangement; it can be crucial. Along with the medical interventions I've mentioned, oral nonsteroidal anti-inflammatories and even injections of lidocane and steroids, yoga may be the key to relieving your pain.

1. FLOATING TADASANA
Floating Mountain

BENEFIT: Promotes realignment of SI joint.

CAUTION: Use soft or thick chair backs (unlike those pictured) to avoid wrist injury or carpal tunnel syndrome.

PROPS: Two chairs.

NOTE: This pose can also be done while sitting in an armchair.

FLOATING TADASANA MODIFIED
AND REGULAR Put two chairs back to
back, far enough apart so that you can
stand comfortably between them.
Keeping elbows straight, press the
heels of the hands onto the tops of the
chair backs. Bend the knees slightly so
that some weight is transferred from
your feet to your hands. Relax abdominal muscles. This release of tension in
the stomach muscles is crucial to doing
this pose successfully. Without that
relaxation, the pose will not work to
relieve SI joint pain.

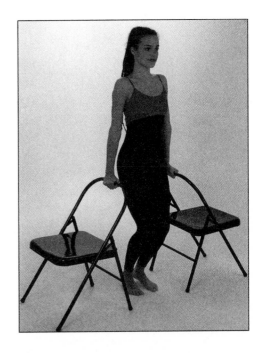

Allow gravity to pull your hips
down while you hold your chest up.
This enables the SI joints to readjust.
Keep abdominal muscles soft, and
relax your back muscles as much as possible. Breathe normally for
ten to fifteen seconds. This pose may be repeated any number of
times during the day. You don't need to do it on an empty stomach.

To come out of the pose, gradually bend your elbows and
straighten your knees.

2. VERTICAL DANDASANA
Vertical Staff

BENEFITS: Realigns SI joint in all three dimensions.

CAUTION: Use a chair with broad arms.

NOTES: When you are in a stable position in this pose, you can
move your torso from side to side and from front to back; you can
also use your shoulders to revolve clockwise and counterclockwise.
That is the three-dimensional element that helps realign the joint
and relieve pain.

This pose is good for office workers; you may be able to do it at
your desk.

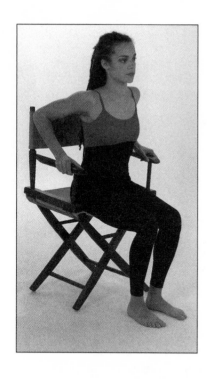

VERTICAL DANDASANA MODIFIED Sit comfortably in a chair, with your forearms and palms on the chair arms and your back straight. Look directly ahead. Move palms back so they are in line with your hips and shoulders. Press down on your palms and straighten your elbows a little to take some of the weight off your buttocks. Keep your feet on the floor. Relax your stomach and back muscles. Let gravity pull your hips down. Breathe with your mouth closed for ten to fifteen seconds. Repeat as often as you wish.

To exit this pose, lower yourself to a sitting position.

VERTICAL DANDASANA REGULAR Begin as above. Straighten your elbows enough so that you raise your buttocks about an inch off the seat. Your feet may be on the floor, but do not put any weight on them. Breathe with your mouth closed for up to half a minute. Experiment with slightly inclining your torso to the right and left, forward and back and rotating it clockwise and counterclockwise. By working with combinations of these movements you may feel a dull or intense ache in the lower back, and then a significant to total relief from pain.

To exit this pose, lower yourself to a sitting position.

3. BHARADVAJASANA
Father of a major character in the *Maharabata*

BENEFITS: Opens SI joints one at a time; improves range of motion in lumbar spine, which reduces stress on SI joints.

CAUTION: Do not do this pose after having total hip replacement surgery.

PROP: Blanket.

BHARADVAJASANA MODIFIED Sit comfortably on the floor with your knees bent. Bring both legs to the right, bending the knees farther. You will be sitting on your left hip joint. Bring your right hand behind you and to the left. Slide your left hand, palm out, along your right thigh and toward the floor. Bring your shoulders back. The top of your chest moves slightly forward and up. Relax the muscles of the abdomen, pelvis, and thighs. Breathe with your mouth closed for ten to fifteen seconds.

To exit this pose, bring your right hand to your side as you take your left hand away from your right thigh. Repeat on the opposite side.

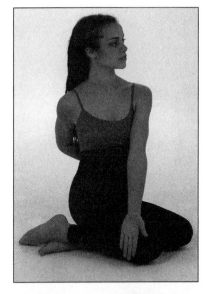

BHARADVAJASANA REGULAR Begin as above but tuck your left hand under your right thigh. Bend your right elbow, reach behind you and grasp your left biceps. Your spine must be quite straight to do this, even though it is turned to the right. Bring both shoulder blades down and together. Raise the upper chest and pull in your stomach. Breathe with your mouth closed for ten to fifteen seconds.

To exit this pose, release your left biceps and bring your right hand to your side. Take your left hand from under your right thigh. Return to a normal sitting position. Repeat, bringing both legs to the left.

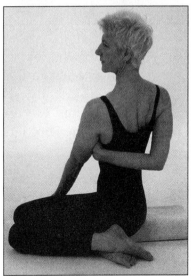

4. GARUDASANA
Eagle

BENEFIT: Stretches connective tissues and muscles of entire back.

CAUTION: If you have had hip surgery less than a year ago, do not do this pose.

PROP: Stable card-table chair.

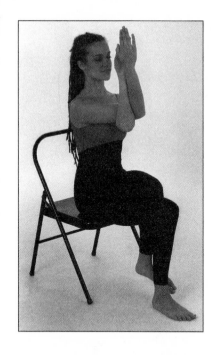

GARUDASANA MODIFIED Sit in a chair with your feet flat on the floor. Cross your left thigh over your right thigh. Hook your left foot behind the right calf. Slide back in the chair, get comfortable, and relax. By slightly extending your left knee you can pull your left thigh farther to the right, opening the left SI joint. Hold for ten to fifteen seconds.

To exit this pose bring your palms to the chair seat or beside your hips. Release your ankle. Return to a normal sitting position. Then do the pose on the other side. This pose may be done from the standing position if strength and balance permit.

GARUDASANA REGULAR While in the modified pose, bend your elbows and raise them so they are at chest level. Put your right elbow into the crook of your left elbow. Bring your hands together and interlace your fingers. Breathe evenly for ten to fifteen seconds.

To exit the pose, bring your palms down to the chair seat beside your hips. Release your ankle and hips. Return to a normal sitting position. Repeat the pose on the opposite side.

5. MAYURASANA
Peacock

BENEFITS: Uses gravity to readjust SI joint. Strengthens abdominal muscles and back extensor muscles.

CAUTION: Doing this pose may cause injury to your ribs if you have severe osteoporosis. Avoid doing this pose if you have gastric reflux syndrome or extreme hypertension. The modified version of this pose is safe for pregnant women; do not do the regular version of this pose if you are pregnant or have carpal tunnel syndrome. The regular version is only for chronic sacroiliac joint derangement. It is nearly impossible to do in the acute stage.

PROP: You may want to use a chair or block or thick book for support for the regular pose.

MAYURASANA MODIFIED Stand close enough so that you are almost touching a kitchen counter, desk, chair, or object of comparable height. Your feet should be comfortably apart. With palms facing away from your body, fingers pointing down, lean forward slightly until the heels of your hands come to rest against the edge of the chair. As you lean forward, dig your elbows into your lowest ribs so that your forearms support of much of but not all of your weight. Your legs do less weight bearing as you lean forward and your heels lift slightly off the floor. Relax your abdomen. You will know you are doing this pose correctly if you feel a stretch or dull ache in your lower back. Keep your abdominal muscles relaxed. Do not move your elbows. Breathe quietly for ten to fifteen seconds.

To exit this pose, gradually straighten your elbows and return your heels to the floor. Release your hands.

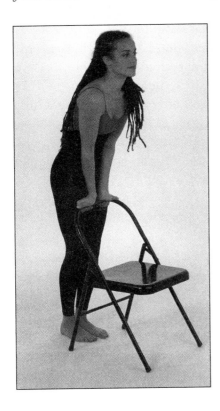

MAYURASANA REGULAR Kneel on all fours with fingertips facing knees. Bring elbows in so they press against the lower ribs, and elbows support your torso. Place the top of your head on the floor. You now have five points of support. Lift and extend your right leg so that it is parallel to the floor. Balancing carefully, extend your left leg so that it is parallel to the right leg. Raise your head so it

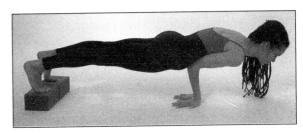

is in line with the rest of your body. Your hands are now the major points of support. Breathe through your nose. Hold the pose for ten to fifteen seconds.

To come out of this pose, bring your left knee to the floor; then bring your right knee to the floor.

6. MARICHYASANA III
Son of Brahma, Creator of the Universe

BENEFITS: Helps rotate joints into proper position.

CAUTION: Do not do this pose during pregnancy.

PROP: Blanket.

MARICHYASANA MODIFIED Sit on a blanket on the floor with your legs extended in front of you. Bend your left knee and bring your left heel close to the perineum and the foot alongside the right thigh. The left shin should be firm and vertical, the right knee straight. Balance your weight evenly on your sit bones. Bend your right arm and revolve your torso counterclockwise until the outside of your forearm and upper arm are flush with the outside of the bent left knee.

Walk your left fingertips behind you and to the right. Use a little pressure against the outside of the left knee to revolve the torso even farther. Keep your shoulders horizontal and your spine straight. Bring your right chest forward and to the left and your left shoulder back and to the right. Breathe quietly for ten to fifteen seconds.

To get out of this pose, release both hands and return to a normal sitting position. Release your left leg carefully. Now reverse your legs and do the pose on the other side.

MARICHYASANA REGULAR Sit on the floor with your legs extended in front of you. Bend your left knee and bring your left heel close to the perineum, the foot parallel to the right thigh and in contact with it. The right foot should be firm and vertical, the right knee straight. Balance your weight evenly on your sit bones. Bend your right arm beyond ninety degrees and revolve your torso counterclockwise until the outside of your right upper arm is in contact with the outside of the bent left knee. Slide the right arm as far as possible beyond the left knee until the back of the right armpit is against it.

Walk your left fingertips behind you and to the right. Bend the right elbow more as you rotate the arm inward, bringing the hand back toward you on the right side of the left shin. Walk even farther behind and to the right with the left fingertips to revolve the torso even more. Then bend your left elbow, bringing it forward toward the right hand. Reach backward and to the right with the right hand. Arch your back to permit the left hand to come forward and grasp the right wrist. Keep your shoulders horizontal and spine straight. Breathe slowly and symmetrically, inflating and deflating both lungs equally for ten to fifteen seconds. To accomplish this pose, begin by bringing the back of the right armpit as close as possible to the outside

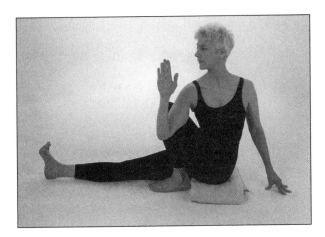

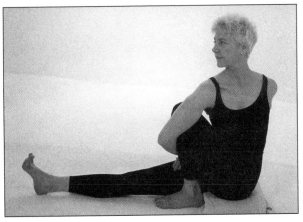

of the left knee. However, keep the right shoulderblade back to improve your leverage and the pose. Now use your left hand to turn your torso more. The right side of your chest comes forward and to the left; the left shoulder goes right and back. Arch your back to permit your left hand to come forward and grasp the right hand more firmly. Breathe slowly and deeply for fifteen seconds.

To get out of this pose, release both hands and return to a normal sitting position. Release your left leg carefully. Repeat the pose with the left leg bent.

There are some poses that are described and pictured elsewhere in the book for other diagnoses that may also be helpful for sacroiliac joint complaints. These poses are, in order of acute to chronic pain:

ANANTASANA—Vishnu's Couch

SUPTA PADANAGUSTHASANA—Holding Big Toe While Supine

ARDHA PADMA PASCHIMOTTANASANA—Half Lotus Forward Bend

BADDHA KONASANA—Bound Angle

CHAPTER 10

Pregnancy

CAUTION: Throughout this book I have identified poses that should not be done if you are pregnant. Please read the cautions and warnings before doing any yoga pose that is not in this chapter. At the same time, I have indicated which poses should be done with care and which ones are perfectly all right. The photographs in these pages show my own version of every pose. Do the poses pictured here, but understand that there are other interpretations and other versions, and those may not be safe, even though they have the same name.

Let me state the obvious: When you're pregnant, you gain weight. The baby forms and is carried in front of you. Taking the baby with you wherever you go requires support, which your back supplies. The baby really puts your back to work. When walking or standing the added weight you're carrying causes your back to arch more than it does when you aren't pregnant. This may cause your shoulders to slump. All this is a recipe for back pain. In addition, all the muscles supporting you—your back, your buttocks, your legs—get tired after a long day's work of carting around the baby. It's important to work to maintain good posture. It's one of the basics for avoiding back pain during pregnancy.

Another factor that may be connected with back pain during pregnancy is blood volume. Physicians, especially in Europe, believe that some of the increased blood supply during pregnancy enters the spinal canal, raising the pressure on the nerves there, which of course can cause trouble.[1] Those who subscribe to this idea and who are knowledgeable about yoga recommend inverted poses as a way to find relief from back pain, and I think that done carefully these poses, including the headstand, are certainly safe for women who regularly do yoga. These can be done right up to the last weeks of pregnancy.

Estimates about how many pregnant women have back pain run as high as 70 percent. This may be back pain that has never occurred before and never will again. Still back pain and pregnancy are a common and difficult combination. For one thing, pregnancy and most medications don't mix. For another, it's considered unwise during pregnancy to have many of the standard diagnostic tests such as X rays and MRIs. This makes both diagnosis and treatment by conventional means problematical. The medical specialty called Physical Medicine and Rehabilitation and yoga offer methods of choice for diagnosis and treatment.

Last we must recognize the hormonal aspect of pregnancy. The placenta secretes Relaxin, which, as its name suggests, relaxes ligaments and other connective tissue, before but especially during the childbirth process. When doing yoga during your pregnancy, you might find that your body is more flexible because of the Relaxin your body is manufacturing. I urge you not to take advantage of this increased elasticity by pushing yourself too far in yoga or elsewhere. If you find that you are able to get into a position that would have been difficult before you were pregnant, do it with extreme caution. But there is a less positive aspect to Relaxin: The overarched lumbar spine and the overburdened sacroiliac and hip joints with looser ligaments are a setup for sacroiliac and vertebral joint dysfunction, which are major sources of back pain in pregnancy.

If you have mild low back pain, it's probably from carrying around fifteen or twenty extra pounds in front of you. I would suggest strengthening back muscles, but carrying the progressively greater weight for months takes care of that. For the back pain, stretching the vertical muscles in your back on either side of your spine should help.

Hip problems that occur during pregnancy can be transitory or serious. If the pain increases with weight bearing or moving the leg and seems to be coming from the hip, ask your doctor before doing yoga.

Then there's the last problem of pregnancy for which yoga may also be perfectly suited: sleep. When the already tired pregnant woman retires, respite may not be easy! The added weight and its distribution often require special new sleeping positions and prohibit the old favored ones. If you are used to sleeping on your back, you might be out of luck because the weight of the fetus and fluids may press down on the back and on spinal nerves, causing pain. Also, as the baby grows, his or her head can press against the lower spine and sacrum, where nerves exit the spine and travel through the intersection called the lumbosacral plexus—another cause of pain. Night may also bring leg cramps.

First, learn what sleeping positions are comfortable through trial and error, and I advise using as many bed pillows as you need to for support. Yoga stretches are wonderful for cramps. Do not hesitate to read up on how to meditate. A good place to begin is with the book, *The Heart of Meditation* by Sally Kempton.[2] Meditation may help you prepare for sleeping at night, and may help with going back to sleep if you wake up because you need to go to the bathroom.

Yoga meditation and breath control will stand you in good stead all through your pregnancy and through the childbirth process. Meditation is valuable for quelling the jitters and for relieving anxiety that accompanies pregnancy, especially a first pregnancy. It will be useful for achieving the calm necessary for a good night's rest.

Breath control is part of yoga meditation, and when you go into labor you will find that there is good reason that a combination of breath control and meditation is at the core of the time-tested Lamaze Method. Breath control helps you master your pain and your reaction to pain, as well as helping you maintain calm and directing thoughts to a secure and confident inner place.

1. Upavistha Konasana
Seated Angle

Benefits: Stretches hamstrings and adductor muscles, improves circulation to pelvic area. This pose is also good for most pain related to sciatica.

Warning: If you have sacroiliac joint derangement, do not do this pose.

Props: Two yoga straps and a blanket

Upavistha Konasana Modified Sit on the floor, back straight, legs spread apart as much as possible. Your spine is erect and your weight should be evenly distributed on the sit bones. You may be more comfortable sitting on a blanket than on the bare floor. Take a breath in. Keeping your back straight, lean forward as you exhale and place your hands on your knees, shins, or ankles as far down as you can. Breathe quietly for ten to fifteen seconds. As you inhale, rise to your original sitting position.

Upavistha Konasana Regular Same as above. Grasp the outsides of your heels or use straps to maximize the forward stretch.

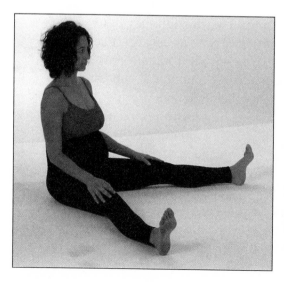 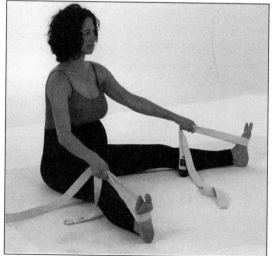

2. BADDHA KONASANA II
Bound Angle

BENEFITS: Good for entire urinary tract. Relieves sciatica by reducing lumbar lordosis (overarching). May minimize tendency to develop varicose veins by maximizing venous drainage.

CAUTION: Do not do this pose if you have sacroiliac joint derangement, because the pose temporarily closes the sacroiliac joints.

BADDHA KONASANA II MODIFIED Sit on the floor with weight evenly distributed on sit bones. Thighs are apart, feet are together. Back is straight. Bring the outsides of your knees down toward the floor. Keeping your back straight, lean forward and place your palms on the floor in line with your shoulders. Crawl forward with your fingertips if possible. When you have gone as far forward as you can, hold that position. Relax the inner thighs and outer buttocks. You can press your elbows into the crevices between your calf and thigh to lower your knees still farther. Breathe quietly for ten to fifteen seconds. Walk fingers back; return to the original position.

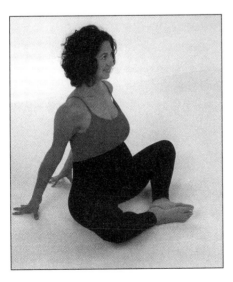
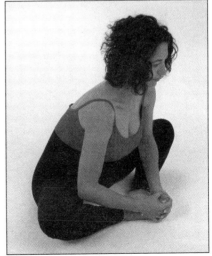

BADDHA KONASANA REGULAR Sit on the floor. Bring heels together and as close to your perineum as possible. Press your knees out and toward the floor. Interlock your fingers around the soles of the feet. Breathe in and, as you exhale, bring your navel down to your heels. Your knees come as close as possible to the floor. Hold the pose for ten to fifteen seconds.

To exit, inhale as you slowly raise your torso.

3. TRIANGA MUKHAIKAPADA PASCHIMOTTANASANA
Three Limbs Placing Face to Leg in West Pose
(literal translation),
or Half Hero

BENEFITS: Reduces low back pain by stretching muscles in spasm. Reduces lumbar lordosis (overarching). Helps knee and hip coordination critical for efficiently carrying baby.

CAUTION: Use several pillows or cushions if you have knee problems.

PROPS: Pillows or cushion and yoga strap.

TRIANGA MUKHAIKAPADA PASCHIMOTTANASANA MODIFIED Sit with a cushion under the right buttock. Extend left leg. Bend the

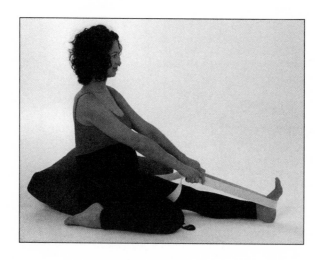

right knee and fold the leg under so that the heel is in line with the hip but off the pillow. Thighs should be parallel, with your right shin at a slightly outward angle. Put your hands on the floor at your sides. Carefully bring your whole torso forward, keeping the left leg and back straight. Move the hands forward as your torso comes forward so that your arms continue to support you. When you have come forward enough to stretch your hamstrings, the lower back, and the muscles that will work during the birth process, hold that position for ten to fifteen seconds. Keep your weight evenly distributed on the sit bones, right shin, and left leg and heel.

Gradually crawl the fingertips back to your sides to exit the pose. Reverse.

TRIANGA MUKHAIKAPADA PASHIMOTTANASANA REGULAR The modified and regular versions of this pose differ only in the placement of the heel. In the regular version the foot is beside the thigh, permitting both sit bones to reach the floor. With this difference, the two poses proceed the same way.

4. SUPTA PADANAGUSTHASANA
Holding Big Toe While Supine

BENEFITS: Relieves low back pain by stretching hip extensor muscles. Reduces sciatica, increases hip joint flexibility, drains blood from legs.

CAUTION: May raise blood pressure slightly (less than ten points).

PROPS: Two pillows and a yoga strap.

SUPTA PADANAGUSTHASANA MODIFIED Lie on the floor with two cushions supporting your back, heels stretched out straight away and far from hips. Your head is stretched away from your shoulders. Raise your left leg, with the knee bent. When the thigh is vertical, straighten your knee. Bring your leg as close as you can to vertical. Grasp your leg with your left hand where you can, as close to the heel as possible. Alternatively, loop a strap around the foot and hold it in the left hand. It is also possible to hold the strap with both hands, but remember, keep your shoulders flat against the pillows. You may use a strap across the bottom of the left foot. Keep your right foot relaxed on the floor. Relax your neck and the abdominal and pelvic musculature. Hold for ten to fifteen seconds, breathing evenly.

To exit the pose, release the hand, bend the knee, and then gradually lower the leg. Repeat the pose on the other side.

SUPTA PADANAGUSTHASANA REGULAR Lie stretched out on your back as in the modified pose, heels stretched out straight and far from your hips. Your head is stretched away from your shoulders, lengthening the neck. Raise the left leg toward vertical, with the

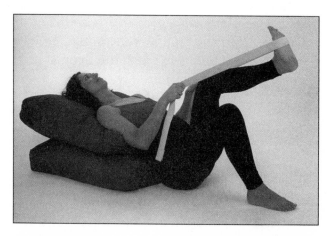

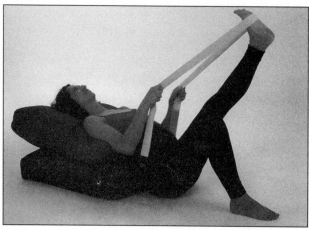

knee bent, until you can either grasp the big toe with the left thumb and first two fingers or loop a belt around the sole of the foot. Then straighten the knee as you raise the leg to vertical. Lie flat, keep the right side relaxed on the floor and both shoulders flush against it. Relax your neck and abdominal and pelvic musculature. Hold for fifteen to thirty seconds.

To exit the pose, release the hand or the belt slowly as you bend the knee and then gradually lower the leg. Repeat the pose on the other side.

5. Gomukhasana
Cow Face

Benefits: Good for leg cramps, sacroiliac joint problems, and upper back pain and stiffness.

Warning: Do with care if you have knee problems.

Props: Two blankets or pillows.

Gomukhasana Modified Sit on floor on two blankets or pillows with legs straight in front of you. Bend your right knee so you are sitting with your right heel under the left thigh and beside your left hip joint. Use your hands to bring your left leg over your right leg. Your left heel should now be beside your right hip joint. Knees will be in line vertically. Bring your right hand, wrist, and forearm behind your head. Press your head back against your forearm to stretch your right armpit. Keep your left hand unengaged to help with balance. With your back straight and chest open, breathe quietly for ten to fifteen seconds.

To leave the pose, use your left hand for balance. First return your right arm to your side, then use your hands to lift your left leg and return it to the floor. Reverse the legs and arm and repeat the pose on the other side.

Gomukhasana Regular Legs and right hand are in position as in the modified pose with blankets or pillows. Bring your left hand around behind you and reach up until you can grasp your right

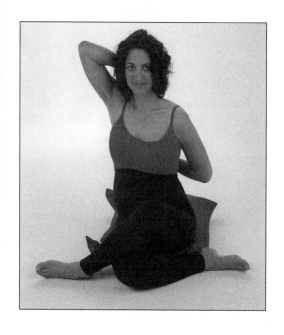

hand. Open your chest. Breathe quietly for ten to fifteen seconds.

When exiting the pose, release your hands first. Then, using your hands to guide your leg, place your right heel in front of you. Use your hands to balance as your left leg releases. Reverse and do the pose on the other side, using legs and arms in the opposite positions.

6. ANANTASANA
Vishnu's Couch

BENEFITS: Relieves low back pain by stretching hamstring and quadratus lumborum muscles. Reduces sciatica, increases hip joint flexibility, drains blood from legs. Increases range of motion for leg movement out to the side (adductors and internal rotators).

CAUTION: May raise blood pressure slightly (less than ten points).

PROPS: Blanket, pillow, and yoga strap.

ANANTASANA MODIFIED Lie on your right side with your right arm supporting your head. Bend your left knee and bring your left leg toward your chest. Hold the left big toe with the index and middle finger of your left hand, or loop a strap around your foot at the arch. You can use a wall behind you for balance. Breathe quietly for ten to fifteen seconds. Then reverse and do the pose on the other side.

To exit, bend your knee as you bring your thigh down to the floor, and release your big toe.

ANANTASANA REGULAR Start in modified pose. Then, keeping your body on the right side and holding your left big toe with your left thumb and fingers or a strap as before, straighten your left leg as

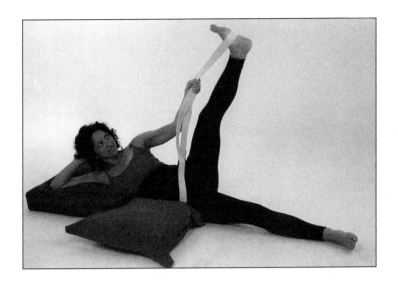

it comes to the vertical. Keep your hip joints perpendicular to the floor. Hold this position for ten to fifteen seconds.

Bend your knee as you come out of the pose, using your right hand for balance. Release the toe. Reverse and do the pose on the other side.

There are some poses that are described and pictured elsewhere in the book for other diagnoses that may also be helpful for backache during pregnancy. These poses are listed in order of acute to chronic pain:

VIRABHADRASANA II—Warrior Pose II

PARSVOTTANASANA—Stretching of the Flank

VIPARITA KARANI—Inverted Lake

VIRASANA—Hero Pose

CHAPTER 11

Spinal Stenosis

Spinal stenosis is a condition in which the spinal canal—the space inside the bony ring of the backbone—narrows. When it involves low back pain, this narrowing generally occurs at the lower end of the lumbar spine, in the central canal, not the exit point of the nerves that serve the entire body below. If these nerves (called nerve rootlets in the lumbar spine) are compressed in a space that is uncomfortably narrow or a tight fit, there is pain.

This pain is neurological in character. That is, it's tingling, shooting, and/or burning. There is frequently numbness, a pinching feeling, or strange sensations—feelings of hot and cold and other unpleasant sensations far away from the root of the nerve that is injured. For example, a nerve root that exits the spine at L5 and is compressed above may cause burning at the outside of the calf and pain between the first and second toes.

The causes of spinal stenosis include arthritis, where the bones become thicker with the accumulation of years, reducing the space inside the spine. Herniated disc is also a cause of stenosis. In that case the room inside the spinal canal is occupied by disc material and the inflammation it brings. Horizontal sliding of the vertebrae, spondylolisthesis, is a third cause of this condition. Actually, anything that narrows the space within the spine produces stenosis, which means "narrowing."

To complicate matters, there's a large ligament just behind these nerves, called the Ligamentum Flavum, which can swell for a variety of reasons, including overactivity, arthritis, autoimmune disease, and other reasons we don't yet understand. Some experts believe that when blood volume goes up quite a bit and hormones change during pregnancy, stenosis can also occur.

You might think that the pain or sensations or lack of them would always be symmetrical because when the space inside your spinal canal is too narrow, everything inside it should be equally compressed. That's generally true. If you have numbness in your left calf, you might very well also have it in your right calf. But it isn't always the case. A disc may herniate to one side and not the other, arthritis can be worse on that side than the other, and inflammation can also take place in localized areas. So, if symptoms hit only one leg, that doesn't necessarily rule out stenosis.

Stenosis is one of those conditions that develops and worsens with age, but there are treatment options. Yoga works in several ways. All the poses I've included in this chapter do the same basic thing. They stretch out the nerves. Increasing the length of the course of a nerve by arching the back, for example, thins the nerves just as stretching a rubber band thins it. Stretching the nerves and all the accompanying adjacent membranes helps them fit better into the spinal canal.[1] One of the poses here, the headstand, also shunts the blood supply from the abdomen and lower back up toward the chest and head. The main thing this does is draw the blood away from your lower back, where there may be too much, especially in pregnancy. But it also has many other benefits, including improving awareness and increasing balance and producing calm.

The poses that follow also strengthen the muscles of the lower spine, which will help the nerves stretch by keeping the back a little more arched. Since the shortest distance between two points is a straight line, curving the lower back increases the distance the nerves must span. The poses increase the distance the nerves have to travel, effectively thinning them so they fit better in the limited space available. Physically stretching the nerves also tends to move them within the canal, reducing the effects of any adhesions. This is good in itself as well as affording this nervous tissue more mobility to enable it to wriggle out of harm's way in a tight situation.

Surgery is often needed for severe spinal stenosis, but I find that medicines—oral and injected steroids and others—in conjunction with yoga are extremely valuable. The poses in this chapter are safe but may produce some inflammation at first, because of their efficacy: moving bones, mobilizing joints, and stretching nervous tissue. If inflammation should occur, mild over-the-counter anti-inflammatory or prescription medicines, including COX-2 inhibitors for people with gastritis, ulcers, or allergies, will likely be helpful. They will probably be unnecessary after a week or two.

1. SALABHASANA I
Locust

BENEFITS: Strengthens extensor muscles, stretches and thins nerves; excellent for keeping spine elastic and abdominal muscles strong.

WARNING: Do not do this pose if you are pregnant or if you have gastroesophageal reflux disorder (GERD).

SALABHASANA I MODIFIED Lie facedown on the floor. Your arms are at your sides, palms facing inward. In this version, the legs are separated and the knees are bent so the shins are vertical. Elevate your thighs and head, using the backs of your hands to help attain more elevation. Then stretch your arms out behind you horizontally and parallel to each other.

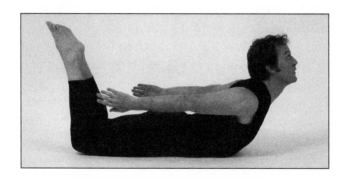

This pose is good for acute back pain. Hold for fifteen seconds. Oppose the tendency to take short, shallow breaths. Breathe slowly and deeply, filling the lungs with air.

To come out of the pose, lower your head and thighs at the same time.

SALABHASANA I REGULAR Lie face down on the floor. Your arms are at your sides, palms facing inward. Legs are together. Raise your head and heels equally from the floor as high as possible. Look up. Arms and hands rise with shoulders and are horizontal.

Hold this pose for fifteen seconds, breathing slowly and deeply, drawing air into the bottom, front, back, and top of both lungs.

Exhale as you slowly lower your feet, head, and arms to their original positions.

2. SALABHASANA II
Locust

BENEFITS: Intensive strengthening of spinal muscles; increased abdominal control.

WARNING: Same as Salabhasana I.

PROP: Folded blanket.

SALABHASANA II MODIFIED Lie on the floor on your stomach with your palms beneath your shoulders, facing down. Press gently on your palms. Keeping your knees straight, raise your thighs, chest

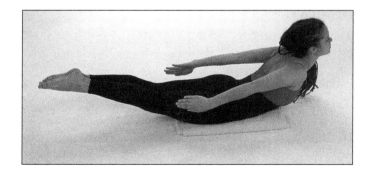

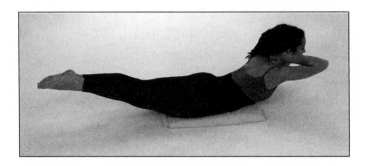

and head as high as possible off the floor. Extend your arms in front of you as far and as high as possible, palms down. Breathe quietly and deeply for ten to fifteen seconds.

To exit the pose, exhale as you bring your hands to their original position beneath the shoulders. Smoothly lower your chest and thighs, then head and legs, using your hands for support.

SALABHASANA II REGULAR Lie on the floor on your stomach. Interlock your fingers behind your head. As you inhale, raise your straight legs, head, and chest as high as possible. Breathe quietly and deeply for ten to fifteen seconds.

To get out of the pose, lower your chest, head and legs. Then bring your hands to your sides.

3. URDHVA DHANURASANA
Upward Bow

BENEFITS: Lengthens lumbar nerve rootlets, thinning them so they are less compressed by the spinal canal. Strengthens extensor muscles of the entire back. Increases facet (joints of vertebrae) flexibility.

CAUTION: Do not do this pose if you are pregnant or have spondylolisthesis or severe cervical arthritis.

PROPS: Two pillows or cushions and a mat for the modified version of this pose.

URDHVA DHANURASANA MODIFIED Lie on two pillows or cushions supporting only the lower tips of your shoulder blades. Open

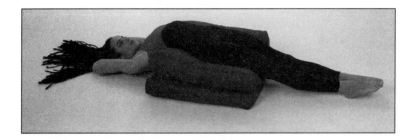

your hips, straighten your knees, point your toes. Fold your arms under your head. Each of these movements should progressively bring your shoulder blades back, together, and downward toward your pelvis. Breathe quietly and slowly for ten to fifteen seconds.

To leave the pose, first unfold your arms and bring your hands to the floor, then relax your legs, bend your right knee, and gently turn over to the left.

URDHVA DHANURASANA REGULAR Begin in the modified position, but without the cushions. Then press down with your palms, straighten your elbows a little, and press down with your feet, straightening the knees somewhat. Arch your back, lift up your chest and pelvis, and arch your back and neck further, so that the top of your head comes to rest on the floor. Hold for fifteen seconds, breathing softly, with your mouth closed.

To leave the pose, bend your knees, tuck in your chin, and bring your head and neck to their normal resting position.

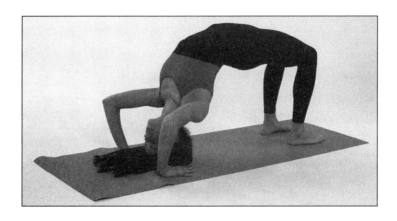

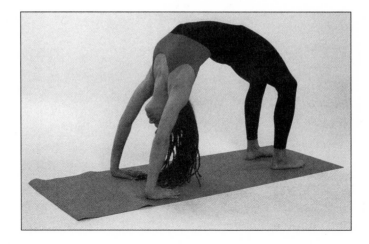

Urdhva Dhanurasana (Advanced) The regular pose can be extended by straightening your elbows fully and your knees somewhat, elevating your head, chest, and navel. Arch your thoracic spine, bring your shoulder blades together, extend your knees as much as possible. Hold this position for fifteen seconds, breathing slowly.

To exit the pose, bend your knees, let your head come down to a resting position, and bring your hands to your sides.

4. Kapotasana
Pigeon

Benefits: Helps stretch lumbar nerves so that they have more room inside the spinal canal. Strengthens extensor muscles of the entire back. Increases the flexibility of the joints associated with the vertebrae.

Caution: Do not do this if you are pregnant, or if you have ankylosing spondylitis. Sit on a pillow if knees are stiff or injured; pillows can also be placed behind you to cushion the upper back and shoulders in the regular pose.

Note: This pose is similar to but not the same as Supta Virasana, Lying-Down Hero (see page 80).

RSASANA MODIFIED (VERSION 1) Place your elbows on the nket about as far apart as your shoulders. Interlock your fingers. s also important to bring the heels of your hands close together. t the crown of your head down at the center of the triangle med by your elbows and hands. Stand up on your toes, straight-ing the knees. Put some weight on your elbows in order to raise ur shoulders. Most of the weight will be on your head.

Walk your feet as close to your head as possible without losing ur balance. Breathe carefully and slowly through your nose for fif-n seconds.

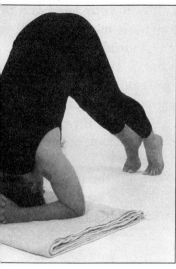

To exit this pose, slowly walk your feet away from your head. Bring your knees to the floor. Supporting your weight on your elbows, bring your head up. Put one palm and then the other on the floor, returning to all fours.

SIRSASANA MODIFIED (VER-SION 2) Begin standing on a car-pet with the backs of your knees a few inches from a chair or couch. Balance your weight evenly on your feet. Move your right leg behind you, bend the knee and put it on the couch or chair seat. Then bend down, also bending your left knee slightly until your hands reach the floor.

Continue to come forward until your palms are on the floor about shoulder width apart. Raise your left leg onto the chair seat. Now both your knees are on the chair or couch behind you. Bend elbows slowly and rest your fore-arms on the floor. Interlock your fingers so that the heels of your

PROPS: Stable card-table chair, pillow.

KAPOTASANA MODIFIED Straddle a folding chair. Place your hands on the top of the back of the chair, bend your right knee and place your foot into the space between the back and the seat of the chair. Then move to the right side of the chair seat, bend the left knee, and insert the left foot into the space between the right foot and the side of the chair. Place both feet squarely on the floor behind the chair, but do not put too much weight on them. (NOTE: If the chair begins to tip, then sit farther from the chair's back. If this still seems unstable, do the pose with a partner who can stabilize the chair for you until you are flexible enough to enter and leave the chair safely.)

Slide your torso farther into the space between the chair back and seat until your buttocks are fully behind the chair. Hold the chair back with both hands and slowly, carefully recline backward, resting the bottom parts of each shoulder blade on the edge of the seat of the chair. Your shoulder blades should be on, not off, the edge of the seat.

Slowly, symmetrically relax the muscles of your throat as you lower your head to a comfortable level. Then release your grip on the back of the chair, place your palms in front of your brow on the floor, fingers pointing toward your heels. Breathe slowly and evenly with mouth closed for ten to fifteen seconds.

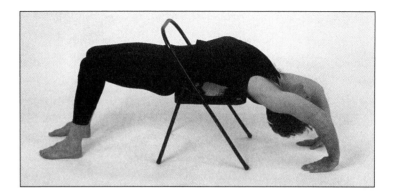

To exit the pose, keep your head and neck extended as you grasp the chair back again and pull your torso up to vertical. Then straighten the head and neck. Slide your hips back some distance out of the chair, but remain in a stable sitting position.

Carefully move your hips to the right and bend your left knee. Raise your left leg, pull it out of the space it's in, and put it on the floor beside the chair. Stand on the left foot, but keep holding on to the back of the chair. Now bring your right foot back until you can put the foot or the knee on the seat of the chair. First regain full balance, then bring your right foot to the floor.

KAPOTASANA REGULAR This begins like the modified version, by straddling a card-table chair. Place your hands on top of the back of the chair; bend your right knee and place your right foot into the space between the back and the seat of the chair. Then move to the right side of the chair seat, bend the left knee, and insert the left foot into the same space as the right. Place both feet stably on the floor behind the chair, but do not put too much weight on them.

NOTE: If the chair begins to tip, then sit out farther from the chair's back. If this still seems unstable, do the pose with a partner who can stabilize the chair for you until you are flexible enough to enter and leave the chair safely. Do not slide your torso farther into the space between the back and seat. Your buttocks should be on the chair, not behind it.

Hold the chair back, slowly sliding both hands farther down the sides as you slowly, carefully recline; shoulder blades are well

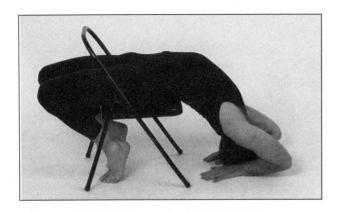

beyond the edge of the seat of the chair. Slowly,
the muscles of your throat as you lower your h
curve it back toward your feet as much as possik

Release the back of the chair; place your pa
brow on the floor, fingers pointing toward your he
back toward your feet with your fingers while y
and bring your feet and toes forward toward
slowly and evenly with mouth closed for ten to fi

To exit the pose, walk your hands back t
before, and straighten your knees to ninety degr
your feet flat on the floor again. Slide your to
space between the chair back and seat. Keep y
extended as you grasp the chair back with both
torso up to vertical. Then straighten the head an

Slide your hips back some distance out of tl
sitting in a stable position. Carefully move your
bend your left knee. Hold on with the right han
leg; pull it back from between the back and seat
it on the floor beside the chair. Stand on the left
to the back of the chair with your left hand.

Bring your right foot back until you can put
on the seat of the chair. First regain full balance
possible dizziness, then bring your right foot to t

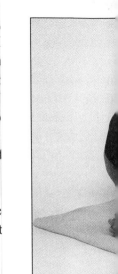

5. APPROACH TO SIRSAS
Headstand

BENEFIT: Relocates venous pool from abdomer

CAUTION: Do not do this pose if you have gl
pressure, cervical disorders or central nervor
dysfunction.

PROPS: Stable card-table and a blanket.

BASIS OF POSE: Go down on all fours. Place
under your shoulders. Knees are together. This
of the next two variations.

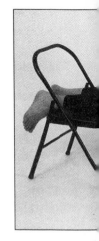

hands are in contact. Rest the top of your head (not your forehead) at the center of the triangle formed by your elbows and hands. Bring your knees forward until your back is vertical. Breathe quietly for ten to fifteen seconds, gradually extending the time over a period of months to five or six minutes.

To exit this pose, release your hands, and one by one replace your palms on the floor just below your shoulders. Then push down with your hands; bring your head up. Slide or creep forward with your hands until there is enough space to bring your left foot down to the floor. Standing on the left foot, slide your hands farther away from the chair until you can bring your right foot to the floor. With knees bent, raise your torso toward vertical. Another way out of this pose is to slide both hands away from the chair, raise the head, and bring the knees one by one off the chair onto the floor. You will be on all fours.

When you no longer have back pain, you will be ready to advance to the full headstand.

6. SAVASANA
Corpse Pose

BENEFITS: Relaxation of all muscles; mental repose.

CAUTION: As Ram Das commented, "One thing about dying, it's completely safe."

PROP: You can use a blanket under your back if it is more comfortable for you than the floor

NOTE: Mr. Iyengar once told me he believes this is the most difficult pose of all.

SAVASANA Lie flat on your back, arms at your sides, palms up. Slide the backs of your hands toward your ankles, bringing your shoulder blades back, down, and together. Stretch your heels away from your hips. Elongate the back of your neck, moving your head as far away from your shoulders as possible. Relax the soft and hard palates inside your mouth. Close your eyes. Breathe smoothly. Hold this pose for one to ten minutes.

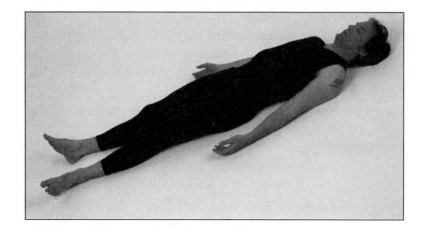

This pose can also be done lying on the floor with the calves supported by the seat of a chair. This way of doing it is invaluable not only for back pain but also for chronic venous insufficiency.

To get out of the pose, open your eyes. Bend your left knee, and roll slowly to the right.

There are some poses that are described and pictured elsewhere in the book for other diagnoses that may also be helpful for spinal stenosis. These poses are, in order of acute to chronic pain:

VIRASANA—Hero Pose

PASCHIMOTTANASANA—West Posture

UTKATASANA—Intense Stretch

CHAPTER 12

Piriformis Syndrome

It's a pain in the butt, often associated with marathon running or marathon sitting in front of the computer, or hours in the car, commuting. Athletes get piriformis syndrome, especially runners, skaters, and dancers. Sometimes this syndrome coexists with other problems, for example, sacroiliac joint derangement, tight hip muscles, hip joint problems, leg-length discrepancy, spondylolisthesis, or herniated disc.

Piriformis syndrome may be the result of an injury suffered in a fall or other trauma. Most often the extreme pain is caused by spasm of the piriformis muscle in the buttock, which compresses the sciatic nerve.

At one time the very existence of piriformis syndrome was in question, and even now there are a few skeptics in the medical profession. However, a few years ago there was a newspaper article in which my research on this problem was published and widely distributed.[1] It led to my seeing many people from inside and outside the United States who had the pain but hadn't known what it was or how to deal with it. Fortunately, those days are behind almost all of them. No pun intended.

Now, with advanced nerve conduction tests, this condition can be identified more easily. Nerve conduction across the tightened piriformis muscle is measurably slowed in stressed positions. This allows for tracking an individual's piriformis syndrome over time, using not only subjective reports of pain intensity, but with objective tests showing that the nerve impulses are gradually picking up speed over time. Since piriformis syndrome has become easier to diagnose and follow, research has been done on treatment efficacy, and treatment has improved. I have found that a combination of medication, physical therapy, and yoga has cured the majority of patients.[2] In a study my colleagues and I published in the *American Journal of Physical Medicine and Rehabilitation*, 90 percent of patients improved 50 percent or more within the first three weeks![3]

The sciatic nerve almost always leaves the buttock below (and rarely, through) the piriformis muscle—a part of human anatomy I compare to the chain guard on a bicycle. Like the chain guard, the piriformis muscle shields the sciatic nerve but isn't important for the motion of the leg.

This muscle is the weakest and least active of the six muscles that abduct and externally rotate the thigh. But it protects the sciatic nerve from injury that comes from sudden movement during sitting and damage from compression by other muscles, against bones or from trauma due to external forces. The piriformis muscle causes trouble when it becomes scarred or tightened and presses against the very nerve it's meant to cushion and protect. A piriformis muscle in spasm squeezes the important sciatic nerve, the largest nerve in the body, causing pain and often altering the function of other muscles further down the leg. But the piriformis muscle's actual function has very little to do with the movement of the bones to which it is attached.

That is why, in rare cases where there must be a last resort, surgery can help piriformis syndrome. The piriformis muscle is routinely cut, removing it from the area of the sciatic nerve, during hundreds of thousands of total hip replacement surgeries that take place every year. These patients have absolutely no ill effects from that aspect of the operation.

Unfortunately piriformis syndrome caused by muscle spasm can become chronic. Once at a Hawaiian luau I was seated next to a neurologist who sat on a special cushion. He carried this cushion with him everywhere he went, and that night he used it as he ate. But even with it, he had trouble remaining seated on the bench. When I asked him what was wrong, it took only a moment for him to confide that he had suffered from piriformis syndrome for fifteen years. His pain was excruciating, his wife confirmed. It was making him miserable, and there seemed no way out. Dinner hadn't started yet. I invited the gentleman to come with me for a few minutes to a secluded spot beneath a tree. There I showed him the Parivrtta Trikonasana, the Twisted Triangle pose. Within five minutes he was feeling enough relief to return to the table, sit down on his cushion, and eat his dinner and dessert without discomfort. Now, to keep acute symptoms from returning, this forty-five year-old physician does just fifteen minutes of yoga every morning before breakfast.

Yoga is an ideal treatment for piriformis syndrome, with one and only one rare exception: If a fall or trauma has scarred the front or edge of the muscle, sometimes stretching won't help. Otherwise, yoga helps by:

- Stretching the muscle and keeping it out of spasm.
- Calming the person and helping relax tension in the piriformis muscle and hip joint.
- Synchronizing coordination and simultaneous muscle contraction that makes it possible to take pressure off the piriformis muscle by improving posture and finding new positions for sitting, walking, and lying down.
- Giving a new bodily outlook that promotes weight loss. Keeping weight down is important because fatty tissue "wads up" and obstructs the path of the sciatic nerve between the hip joint and the ischial tuberosity, narrowing it during sitting and actually contributing to the compression of the nerve.
- Relieving sacroiliac joint dysfunction that frequently plays a key role in spasm of the piriformis muscle.

1. ARDHA MATSYENDRASANA I
Matsyendra was one of the fathers of hatha yoga.

BENEFITS: Asymmetrically stretches tendons, ligaments, and muscles connected to SI joint as well as the piriformis muscle.

CAUTION: Do not do this pose if you are pregnant. Do not push yourself when doing this pose. Beginners risk dislocating rib joints if they push themselves too much. If you have recently had total hip replacement surgery, avoid this pose.

PROP: A blanket can be used for both the modified and regular versions of this pose.

ARDHA MATSYENDRASANA I MODIFIED Sit on the floor. Bend your left knee. Place your left calf under the right knee and the side of your left foot on the floor near your right buttock. Bend your right knee and raise the right leg over the left thigh. Place the sole of the right foot on the floor just beyond your left thigh. Bend your left elbow as you incline your torso forward and to the right. Keeping the elbow bent, slide your left arm as far as possible along the outside of the right knee.

Walk your right fingertips behind you and to the left. Bring the left side of the chest forward and to the right. Bring the right shoulder back and to the left. Turn your torso clockwise. Your shoulders should be parallel with your right leg. Breathe as symmetrically as possible for ten to fifteen seconds.

To exit this pose, release the pressure of your left elbow on your right leg and slide both arms to your sides. Do it on the other side.

ARDHA MATSYENDRASANA I REGULAR Sit on the floor. Bend your left knee and place your left calf under the right knee and your left foot on the floor near your right buttock. Bend your right knee and raise the right foot over the left thigh. Place the sole of your right foot on the floor beside and beyond your left thigh. Your right shin should be vertical. Raise your left arm and slide it outside the right knee so that the back of the armpit gets as close to the knee as possible.

Walk your right fingertips behind you. Bring your left chest forward and to the right. Bring your right shoulder to the left and back.

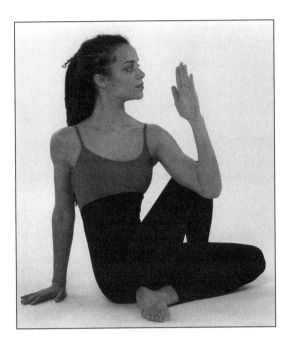 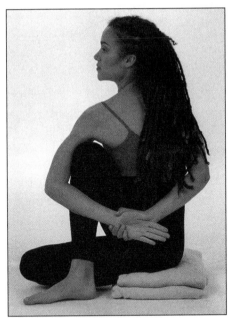

Keep your spine as vertical as possible and twist your torso ninety degrees clockwise. If possible slide your left hand behind your right shin and bring your right hand forward and to the left so you can grasp your left wrist with your right hand. Your shoulders should be parallel with your right leg, and horizontal. Relax all pelvic muscles. Breathe slowly, inflating each lung equally, for ten to fifteen seconds.

To exit the pose, release your grip on the left wrist and slide your arms to your sides. Reverse the legs to do the pose on the other side.

2. PARIVRTTA TRIKONASANA
Twisted Triangle

BENEFITS: Stretches piriformis muscle diagonally, as well as glutei and abductors and external rotators of the thigh and the posterior hip capsule.

CAUTION: Do not do this pose if you are pregnant. Do not do this on a full stomach or after total hip surgery

PROPS: Stable card-table and a mat.

PARIVRTTA TRIKONASANA MODIFIED Stand facing a wall with your feet about three feet apart. Left foot is parallel to the wall. Right foot is at a thirty degree angle with the wall. Stretch your arms out horizontally as far as possible at shoulder height. Turn your entire torso to the left. Keeping your knees straight, bring your right hip forward and your left hip back until the inner thighs are touching. Slide your right arm along the wall, to the left and down until you can grasp your left shin or ankle. You may also use a chair. Now you can horizontally stretch the muscles in the left buttock and the hip joint capsule more by bringing the left part of your back in contact with the wall. If you cannot keep your left arm elevated, place it at your side. Breathe smoothly and symmetrically. Hold the pose for ten to fifteen seconds.

To exit, stretch the arms horizontally while you reverse the twist in the hips and at the same time turn the feet so they are perpendicular to the wall. Step back if you feel off balance. Bring your hands to your sides. Repeat on the other side.

PARIVRTTA TRIKONASANA REGULAR Do the pose without the wall. This requires more balance. Fine points of this more advanced

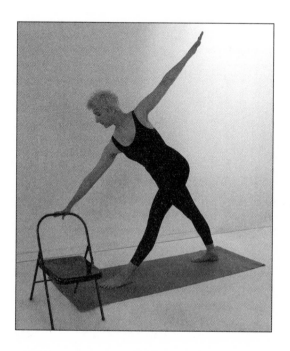

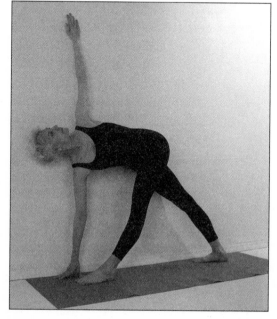

version include attaining the pose and then lengthening the inner thigh of the front leg and equalizing your weight within each foot and between your feet. Breathe as symmetrically as possible for ten to fifteen seconds.

To exit the pose, release your right hand. As you bring your torso to vertical, stretch both arms horizontally and simultaneously return hips and feet to a forward-facing position.

3. PARIVRTTA ARDHA CHANDRASANA
Twisted Half-Moon

BENEFITS: Horizontally stretches piriformis muscle and glutei and abductors and external rotators of the thigh, as well as the hip joint capsule.

CAUTION: Do not do this pose if you are pregnant. Try this against a wall first. Do not do it on a full stomach or after total hip surgery.

PROPS: Two chairs.

PARIVRTTA ARDHA CHANDRASANA MODIFIED Stand with one chair behind you and another chair about two feet in front of you. Stretch out the left leg behind you until the top of the left foot is resting on the chair seat. Place the left hand on the chair in front of you or on the floor (or grasp the leg of the chair), in line with the left

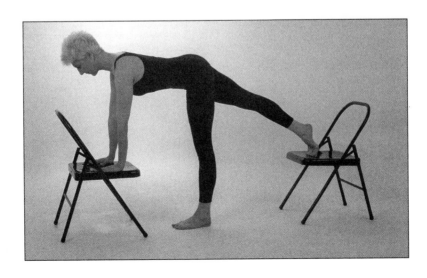

foot. As you do this the entire left side of your body—the shoulder, chest, hip, and leg—should curl downward as much as possible, as shown in the photo.

The right arm should rise, with the elbow straight, in line with and directly above the left shoulder. This position stretches the right buttock quite a bit. Breathe slowly and symmetrically for ten to fifteen seconds.

To exit the pose, raise the left side of your body to the horizontal at the same level as the right. Then bring the left foot back to the floor. Keep your left hand on the chair until then. Return the right hand to your side or use it with the left on the chair seat to balance as you bring your torso back to vertical.

Do the pose on one side, then reverse the legs and do on the other side (pictured above).

Parivrtta Ardha Chandrasana Regular Do the same pose without the wall and with one chair to support your leg. With practice you should strive to become proficient enough doing the modified pose so that you can do the regular pose with at most one chair. As you improve your calm and balance, you may lift the leg off the chair. Some practitioners do not need the chair at all. Hold the pose for ten to fifteen seconds. To exit the pose, lower the horizontal leg to the floor and raise your torso to vertical.

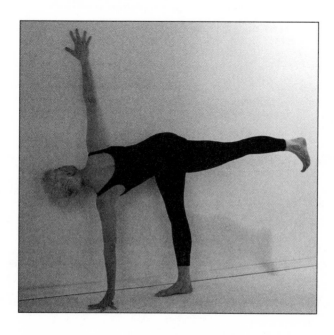

4.VIRASANA
Hero

BENEFITS: Stretches lower back muscles and stretches lateral hip muscles. Stretches soft tissue of back (ilio lumbar fascia). Relaxes iliopsoas and rectus femoris (other hip flexor). Good for pregnant women.

CAUTION: Don't do this pose if you have knee problems.

PROPS: Pillows or blankets.

VIRASANA MODIFIED Sit on a large pillow, knees bent, thighs close to parallel, feet and toes pointing back. Your shins should be outside your thighs but touching the sides of the pillow. Use your hands to pull your calves to the outside so you can sit lower and more comfortably. Arch your back slightly. Try to put your ears, shoulders, hips, and heels in one plane. Open your chest. Place the palms or backs of your hands on your thighs. Keeping your head erect, tuck in your chin. Pull in your stomach. Relax leg, chest, and back muscles. Breathe quietly with your mouth closed for ten to fifteen seconds.

To leave this pose, bring your hands to the floor and kneel on all fours.

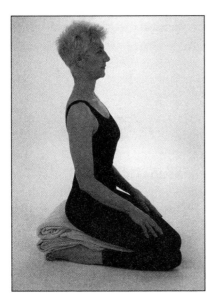
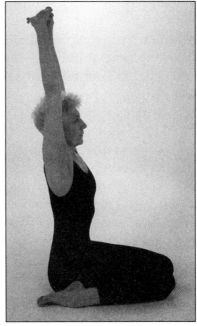

VIRASANA REGULAR To progress in this pose, reduce the size of the pillow you are using until you don't need it anymore. Do not do this too quickly, however, or you could injure your knee. Interlock your fingers and extend them fully overhead, bringing your biceps behind your ears.

Exit as above.

5. EKA PADA RAJAKAPOTASANA I
King of Pigeons

BENEFITS: Stretches buttock musculature. Stretches flexors of the opposite thigh. Balances flexor-extensor mechanism.

CAUTION: Be careful not to exaggerate the arch of the lumbar spine.

PROPS: Chair and mat.

EKA PADA RAJAKAPOTASANA I MODIFIED Kneel with one foot behind a chair or other means of support. Slide your left knee forward as you turn your left shin inward, i.e., toward the right. As you do this, slide your right leg backward. Your torso will descend more and more as the left thigh comes forward and the left leg goes back. As this happens, put your hands and forearms on the seat of the chair for support. Keep your hips parallel to the front of the chair. Your navel should face forward. Shoulders should be even. Breathe quietly for ten to fifteen seconds.

To exit the pose, press down on the seat of the chair with your forearms and pull your left leg back until you are able to slide your right knee forward. You are now in a kneeling position. Repeat on the opposite side.

EKA PADA RAJAKAPOTASANA I REGULAR Kneel, then assume an all-fours position. Advance your left knee toward your left hand, inclining the thigh outward so the shin is in contact with the floor, and the left foot comes closer to the right hand. The pelvis will move forward toward the outstretched hands, and the right leg will end up straighter and farther behind.

Continue to slide the left leg forward and slide your straight right leg backward until your left heel is in contact with your right groin and the outside of the left foot is on the floor. Put your hands at your

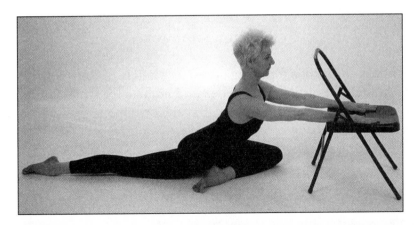

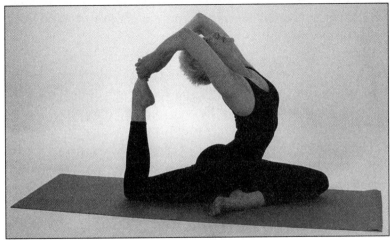

waist, palms facing downward. Arch your entire spine, beginning just above the pelvis. Bring your head back as far as possible. Breathe quietly for ten to fifteen seconds to establish balance. Place your right palm on the floor and bring your left hand over your head as you bend your right knee ninety degrees. Grasp your right foot with your left hand and bring your right hand back to join it. Breathe quietly, being careful to relax unnecessary tension. Hold for ten to fifteen seconds, breathing evenly.

To exit the pose carefully, release the foot and bring both hands to the floor. Straighten your right knee. Bend forward, weight on your palms, and bring the left knee back until you are on all fours. Repeat on the opposite side.

6. JATHARA PARIVARTANASANA
Rolling Stomach

BENEFITS: Stretches piriformis muscle. Stretches hamstrings; vertically stretches buttocks. Stretches and adjusts legs and abdominal fascia and entire digestive system and spleen. Opens sacroiliac joint. Improves lower back range of motion. Strengthens abdominal and lower back muscles.

WARNING: May be painful with spondylolisthesis or herniated disc. Do not do if you have an abdominal hernia.

NOTE: Slowly transition from the modified pose to the regular one by straightening your knees a little more each time you do the pose. You can do this over a period of months.

JATHARA PARIVARTANASANA MODIFIED Lie on your back with arms stretched out horizontally, palms down. Bend your knees. Bring your heels and knees together and the heels as close to the buttocks as possible. Raise your feet off the floor until your thighs are vertical. Keeping your legs together, swing your hips slightly to the left. Then bring your thighs over to the floor on the right. Press your right hand and arm onto the floor to bring your left shoulder flush with the floor. Relax rectal muscles, torso, neck, and shoulders. Breathe with your mouth closed for ten to fifteen seconds.

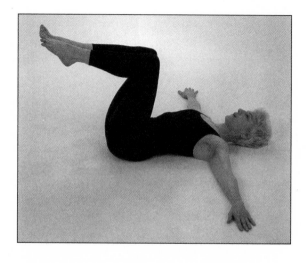

To exit, bring your legs to vertical, lower your thighs until your feet are on the floor. Do this pose on the other side.

JATHARA PARIVARTANASANA REGULAR Lie on your back with arms stretched out horizontally, palms down. Bring your knees and heels together, heels as close to the buttocks as possible. Raise your feet off the floor until your thighs are vertical. Once you are there, straighten your knees until your legs are vertical. Swing your hips a little to the left. Keeping your legs straight and extended, exhale and let your legs descend to the right until they reach the floor. Adjust your hips, if necessary, to keep your heels in line with each other. Pressure on your right palm will bring your left shoulder blade to the floor. Relax rectal muscles. Breathe with your mouth closed for ten to fifteen seconds. Then raise legs to vertical, swing hips to the right and then let the legs descend to the left, using the left hand to lower the right shoulder blade to the floor. Relax rectal muscles, torso, neck, and shoulders. It is best to perform the pose on the other side at this point using the same breathing.

To exit the pose, bring your legs back to vertical, bend your knees, lower your legs to the floor.

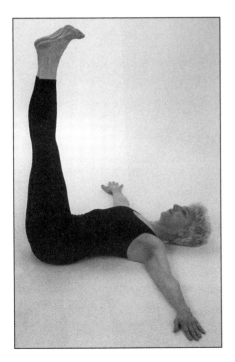

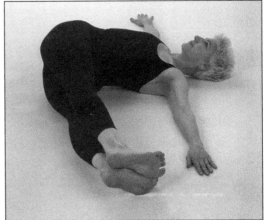

There are some poses that are described and pictured elsewhere in the book for other diagnoses that may also be helpful for piriformis syndrome. These poses are, in order of acute to chronic pain:

GOMUKHASANA—Cow Face

HALASANA—Plow

PASCHIMOTTANASANA—West Posture

JANU SIRSASANA—Head to the Knee Forward Bend

CHAPTER 13

Weight Control

While Western medicine and science concentrate on how the mind affects the body—how we decide to move a finger or turn our heads—yoga puts more focus on feedback from the body to the mind. Signals from the joints, muscles, ligaments, and so on have a great influence on our moods, our impressions of how we feel, our muscle tone, and many other basic elements of our state of being at any given moment. A conscious person becomes more sensitive to these signals through the steady practice of yoga.[1]

It is hardly necessary to mention that one of the signals from body to mind that many people either miss or misread is the one indicating that the stomach is full, or that it is full enough to be satisfied. One reason for this is that many of us just don't pay attention to what our stomachs are telling us. We get the message, but we ignore it and go right on eating. This recreational eating is encouraged by an increase in portion size both at home and in restaurants, by heavy concentrations of fats in many of the foods we enjoy, and by the large amounts of carbohydrates to which we've become accustomed.

In addition, it's important that the stomach is smooth muscle. It is able to expand to contain just about whatever is put into it. Once you have eaten enough to make your stomach larger than it was, then the next time it's empty it sends demands for food to fill it to its greater size. This, of course, becomes a vicious cycle. Too much food expands the stomach, which then needs more for you to feel satisfied than it did before and possibly, though thoroughly filled, it expands further. The waistline quickly follows suit.

When weight stretches out in front of your body, in your arms and torso and certainly in your abdomen, the muscles in your back have to work harder than they would otherwise. If you hold even an egg in its shell out in front of you for long, it becomes heavier and heavier. The same happens when you eat too much and gain weight. The more you gain, the more is stretched out in front of you. This increases both the weight on your spine and the mechanical disadvantage of the spine—the body's axis of support.

Carrying more weight out in front of you makes the muscles of the lower back stronger. Actually it may cause those muscles to become overly strong, disproportionately stronger than the abdominal muscles, which flex the trunk and bend it forward. This imbalance will stiffen the spine to maintain balance and will also make the muscles contract so tightly that one or more may go into extremely painful spasm. This causes other crucial muscles, for example those that help you twist, to become deconditioned through disuse. Actually, all the spinal muscles that aren't working to hold that weight out in front of you, keeping you from toppling forward, may become quite weak, unable to oppose effectively the painful spinal extensor muscles.

Yoga has three solutions: It helps you learn to pay attention to those signals your stomach is sending up to your brain; it helps strengthen spine flexors, abdominal musculature that can limit extensor spasm in the lower back; and it may increase your self-control so that you are able to leave the table, or at least to stop eating, when you're still 5 or 10 percent unsatisfied. Although this may be very slightly uncomfortable at first, you will lose four to five pounds a month, and safely, without risk, without medication, and without counting calories. You can eat anything you want.

The beauty of the simple diet I've outlined above is that your caloric intake will fall, and the size of the organ that is the stomach will gradually decrease. Because your stomach is smaller, you will feel that you require less food. After having followed this routine for a couple of months and losing four to five pounds a month, you will find that your stomach is small enough to make it difficult to regain the weight you have lost so safely and easily.

In addition, almost all the yoga poses, but especially the ones here, help focus the mind on feedback from the body. Conscious pursuit of yoga postures helps you gain the mastery over yourself that makes pushing away from the table before you are full much easier. As time goes on, you will become more aware of your body's internal signals and more able to follow its "instructions."

A secondary problem associated with being overweight is foot pain. Feet are only so big, and although weight may increase, the area of support provided by those two feet will not increase proportionately. Too many pounds per square inch on the bones and soft tissues of the foot often causes difficulties with arches, joints, and ligaments, bruising the bones and causing a lot of discomfort. Simple weight reduction is frequently the answer to foot pain. When a person has lost weight, the pressures on feet come back to normal and they provide support without any pain whatsoever, if being overweight has not previously contributed to deformities.

All yoga poses promote the proper adjustment of weight. Some are particularly beneficial in focusing the mind on the stomach's signals, such as Viparita Karani (4, chapter 6, "Musculoskeletal Pain," p. 72) and Bhujangasana (2, chapter 7, "Herniated Nucleus Pulposis," p. 88).

A number of special factors come into play when a person is trying to control weight. Endurance may decrease. Fatty tissue is quite vascular, yet the size of the heart muscles and their pumping capacity will not rise beyond certain limits, which they reach through steady, vigorous exercise, but not necessarily through the type of yoga poses presented here. Balance may be impaired. Girth may make assuming certain positions difficult.

People who are overweight often have diabetes and physical problems that arise from this condition, such as neuropathy, impaired balance and coordination, pain with exercise, restricted range of motion, and other difficulties. All the poses in these pages are intended for people who are not more than twenty to thirty pounds above their "ideal" weight. Others should consult a clinician before beginning yoga.

1. VIRABHADRASANA I
Warrior I

BENEFITS: Promotes awareness of the stomach (the organ) and of the small intestine. Enhances balance of hip abductors and adductors and strengthens legs. Asymmetrically coordinates internal and external rotators. Improves carriage and back muscle strength, which has the effect of reducing fatty accumulation visible around the hips.

CAUTION: Do not do this pose if you have had total hip replacement surgery or abdominal surgery in the last three months. Do it carefully if you have severe knee problems.

POSSIBLE PROPS: Two stable card-table chairs, placed back-to-back but far enough away from each other so that you can stand between them.

VIRABHADRASANA I MODIFIED You can do this pose as described below: Begin with two chairs (not pictured) back to back, one in front of you and one behind you. Stand with your legs five feet apart. Turn your left foot out ninety degrees and your right foot in thirty degrees. Bring your left hip back and your right hip forward so that your torso is turned counterclockwise ninety degrees and your navel is facing the same direction as your left foot. If you are using chairs, place your hands on the tops of the chair backs. If you are not using chairs, raise your arms over your head until they are vertical. Bend your left knee until you get it as close to a right angle as possible. The right knee stays straight. Keep your torso vertical. Look straight ahead. Breathe with your mouth closed for ten to fifteen seconds.

Continue with your arms in their current position. Then slowly straighten the left knee. If you are using chairs, release your hands. Now turn your left foot in thirty degrees and your right foot out ninety degrees and revolve the torso 180 degrees clockwise, moving the left hip forward and to the right and the right hip backward and to the

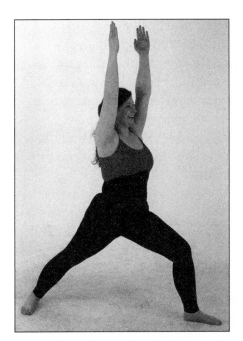 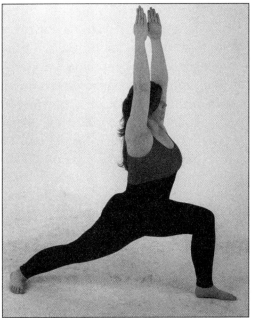

left. To exit the pose, straighten the right knee. Bring your feet to a parallel position. Repeat the pose on the other side.

VIRABHADRASANA REGULAR Stand with your legs five feet apart. Turn your left foot out ninety degrees and your right foot in thirty degrees. Bring your left hip back and your right hip forward so that you rotate your torso ninety degrees counterclockwise, and your navel is in line with your left big toe. Unless you are experiencing severe low back pain, raise your arms to vertical so your biceps are behind your ears and your palms are facing each other. If you have severe low back pain, keep your arms at your sides. Look straight ahead, stretching the entire torso upward, especially the chest, forearms, and thumbs.

Bend your left knee to a right angle. Your shin is vertical and your thigh is horizontal. Pull your stomach in. Keep your torso vertical. Stretch up still farther with your fingertips while your lower body supports you. Breathe with your mouth closed for ten to fifteen seconds. Then, holding the position of your torso and arms, straighten the left knee.

Reverse by turning your right foot out ninety degrees and your left foot in thirty degrees. Revolve your torso 180 degrees clockwise so that the navel is in line with the right big toe. Repeat the process outlined for the left side, bending the right knee to ninety degrees, maintaining an erect torso, with arms stretched upward while breathing with your mouth closed for ten to fifteen seconds.

Following this, to exit the pose, slowly and steadily straighten the right knee and turn the feet and torso to a normal, forward-facing position. Repeat the pose on the other side.

2. VIRABHADRASANA III
Warrior III

BENEFITS: Strengthens extensor muscles of the entire back and legs. Increases awareness of the stomach and small intestine, balances and shapes leg muscles, strengthens shoulder flexor muscles.

CAUTION: Do not do this pose if you have high blood pressure; it may raise your blood pressure ten points or more. Requires a modicum of balance.

PROP: Stable card-table chair.

NOTE: This pose, in its modified and regular versions, begins where Virabhadrasana I ends.

VIRABHADRASANA III MODIFIED Place your chair at your right side three feet beyond your right fingertips. After you have held Virabhadrasana I for ten to fifteen seconds, straighten your left knee by about half. Incline your torso forward to an angle of forty-five degress. Your arms should be a direct extension of your torso. Grasp the chair back as you straighten your left knee completely. Your extended right leg rises until it is in line with your buttocks. Flatten the back of your body as much as possible by lowering the right buttock to horizontal. Use the chair for support. Breathe as normally as possible for ten to fifteen seconds.

To exit this pose, bend the left knee again so that it is close to a right angle. Your torso comes to vertical; your right foot comes back to the floor behind you. Then straighten your left knee. Bring your feet back to parallel. Return to a normal standing position. Repeat on the other side.

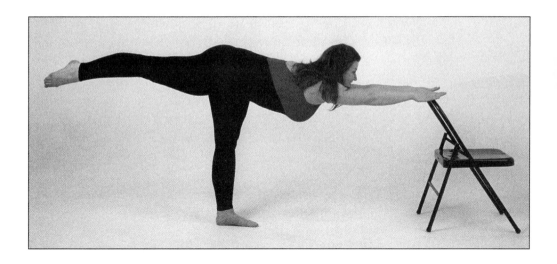

VIRABHADRASANA III REGULAR This also follows from the Regular Virabhadrasana I. After you have completed that pose, breathing in it for ten to fifteen seconds, straighten your left knee by about half. Bring your torso forward and down at a forty-five-degree angle. Keep your arms elevated, parallel, and in the same extended position relative to your torso. Straighten your left knee as you bring your torso forward and down to horizontal. At the same time raise your right leg so that it is in line with your buttocks. Stretch your fingertips forward and your right heel backward. Spread out the toes of your right foot. The whole back of your body should be in a horizontal plane, including the buttocks. This is an arduous but exhilarating pose. Stay as still as possible as you breathe calmly for ten to fifteen seconds. Gradually extend the time you hold the position to a full minute.

To exit the pose, bend the left knee. Raise the shoulders and chest. Keep the right knee straight as you bring the right foot to the floor and bend your left knee to a ninety-degree angle. At the same time raise your torso and arms to vertical. Then straighten your left knee. Bring your feet back to parallel and lower your arms. Return to a normal standing position.

Also, be sure to do Virabhadrasana I and III facing the right side. If time is at a premium, either the modified or regular version of Virabhadrasana I on the right side can lift directly into Virabhadrasana III on the right. Thereafter, Virabhadrasana I on the left side can lift into the left version of Virabhadrasana III. Alternatively, if strength is the goal, it is better to do Virabhadrasana I on both the right and the left, and then repeat that pose on each side as the first part of Virabhadrasana III.

3. PADAHASTASANA
Foot, Hand

BENEFITS: Painlessly brings attention to sensations in stomach and intestine, reducing appetite.

CAUTION: Don't do this pose on a full stomach. Be careful when coming out of this pose to avoid further injury to your back.

PADAHASTASANA MODIFIED Stand with feet parallel and directly beneath hips. Balance your weight evenly on your feet. Take a breath in, opening your upper chest and pulling your shoulders back. Your spine should be slightly concave as you bend forward from the hips. Bring your chest down as close to the floor as possible. Do not hunch your upper back or neck. To avoid doing so, fold your arms in front of your head. Hold for ten to fifteen seconds. Gradually increase the time you hold this pose to half a minute.

Before exiting this pose, let your back and shoulders bend forward a little. Your spine should be slightly convex. Walk your way up your legs with your hands as you raise your torso and return to the standing position.

PADAHASTASANA REGULAR Stand with feet parallel and directly beneath your hips. Knees should be straight. With your back slightly concave, bend forward from your hips, placing your palms on the soles of your feet and the backs of your hands on the floor. To intensify this pose, bend elbows to apply pressure with your palms against the soles of your feet. Find a modestly challenging degree of stretch, hold it, and breathe calmly for ten to fifteen seconds.

Exit as you do in the modified version of this pose, first making shoulders and spine somewhat convex, then releasing your hands and using them to walk up your thighs until you rise to vertical.

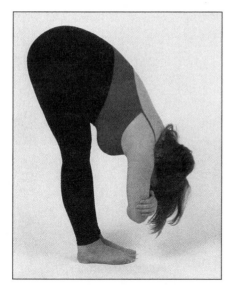 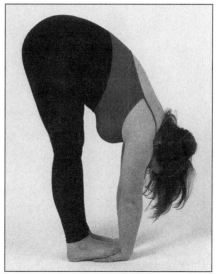

4. ARDHA MATSYENDRASANA (VARIATION)
Sage

BENEFITS: Squeezes and stretches stomach, liver, gallbladder, pancreas and small and large intestines.

CAUTION: Do not do this pose if you are pregnant. Wait four to five hours after eating to do this pose.

PROP: Blanket.

ARDHA MATSYENDRASANA MODIFIED Sit on the floor. Turn your left leg inward and bend the left knee so that the left foot is just in front of the right buttock. Raise your right leg and bend your right knee, lifting the right foot over the left thigh and placing it on the floor. Your right foot is on the floor, shin vertical. Weight is evenly balanced on the sit bones. Grasp the top of your right knee with your left hand. Slide the back of your left arm past the outside of your right knee as far as you can. Walk your right hand behind you, moving your left shoulder back while pulling your left chest toward the right. Keep the spine straight and vertical. Your left arm is like a lever; your right knee is the fulcrum. Do not use it to bring the left shoulder forward, but rather the right chest. Your shoulders should be in line with your right shin.

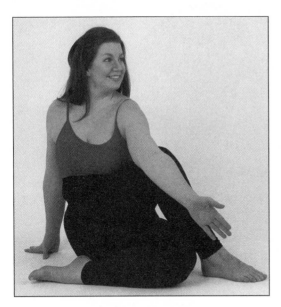 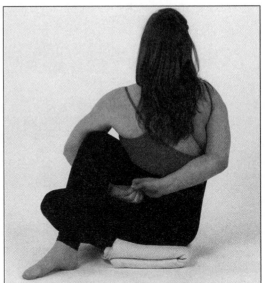

Hold the position for ten to fifteen seconds, inflating the lungs equally as you breathe. It is important to keep your weight balanced on the sit bones during this time.

To exit the pose, gradually release the pressure of the left arm on the knee as you bring your right arm to your side.

ARDHA MATSYENDRASANA REGULAR Sit on the floor. Bend your left knee inward, moving the left foot close to the right buttock. Bend the right knee and raise the right foot over the left thigh, placing the right foot squarely on the floor. Incline the left torso forward and to the right, sliding the outside of the left arm as far as possible forward along the outside of the right knee. Bring the outside and back of the left armpit as close to the outside of the right knee as possible. Tuck your left hand under the right knee and slide the forearm to the left. Walk behind and to the left with right fingertips. Use your right arm to pull your right shoulder back and to the left. Clasp your hands. Use your left arm as a lever to push your left chest forward and to the right. When you have a maximum twist, relax your abdominal muscles. Inflate lungs as symmetrically as possible and breathe evenly for fifteen to thirty seconds.

To exit this pose, release your left hand and bring it, palm down, to the floor beside your left hip. Walk your right fingertips to the right. Inhale as you come out of this pose. Do on the other side.

5. PARIVRTTA JANU SIRSASANA
Twisted Head to Knee

BENEFITS: Increases awareness of sensations from the stomach and duodenum. Tones smooth muscles of the stomach. Stretches hamstrings one side at a time.

CAUTION: Do not do this pose if you are pregnant. Wait five hours after eating to do this pose. Do not do this pose if you have active gastritis or esophageal varices.

PARIVRTTA JANU SIRSASANA MODIFIED Sit on the floor with legs extended in front of you. Bend your right knee and place it on the floor as far to the right as possible. The outside of the ankle, calf, and thigh should be on the floor. The heel is as close to the thigh as possible. Your toes should be touching your left thigh. Turn your torso to the right and extend your left arm. Turning clockwise so the back of your arm is against your left knee, place your right hand on your right thigh. Press against the thigh so that your torso inclines toward the left leg. Slide your left arm forward until you can grasp the top of the left foot with your little finger and the arch of the foot with index finger and thumb. Breathe with your mouth closed for ten to fifteen seconds. It is difficult to breathe slowly in this position, but do your best, while holding your abdominals in.

To exit the pose, slide your right hand to the outside of the right thigh. Release your left hand, placing the left palm on the left shin. At the same time, press up with the left arm and come up to a sitting position. You can pull with your right hand to aid the process. Reverse legs and do the pose on the other side.

PARIVRTTA JANU SIRSASANA REGULAR Sit on the floor with legs extended in front of you. Bend your right knee as much as possible

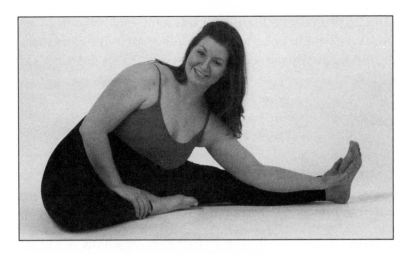

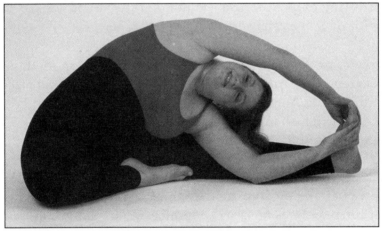

and widen the angle between the right and left thighs to 135 degrees. Turn your torso to the right and revolve your left arm counterclockwise as you extend it along the inner left leg. The outside of the upper arm and deltoid region should be in contact with the inner thigh. Grasp your left big toe with the little finger and the arch of the foot with the thumb and index finger. Use your left elbow to put pressure on the inside of your left knee and rotate your trunk counterclockwise. Bring your back ribs down to the left leg.

Now bring your right arm over your head to grasp the little-toe side of the foot. The little finger is at the top of the foot and the other fingers are closer to the floor. Breathe in and bend your elbows as much as possible. Put pressure on the left knee with the left elbow and pull the right shoulder back, twisting still farther. This is an exhilarating pose. It will be difficult to breathe slowly and impossible to breathe deeply, but try for ten to fifteen seconds.

To exit the pose, release the right hand and then the left hand. Turn your torso to the left as you come to a sitting position. You can support your ascent with your left hand on your left shin, knee, or thigh. Reverse and do this pose on the other side.

6. HALASANA
Plow

BENEFITS: Improves perception of abdominal organs. Stretches buttock musculature and hamstrings. Takes pressure off pudendal nerves in the area between genitals and anus.

WARNING: Do not do this pose if you are pregnant or have glaucoma or hypertension. If you have your period, a full stomach, or shoulder dislocation do not do this pose.

PROPS: Stable card-table chair and one or more blankets

HALASANA MODIFIED (VERSION I) Lie diagonnally with your right hip a few inches in front of the right front leg of a chair. Bend your knees halfway and bring your thighs up until they are vertical. Gradually move your legs up and over to the right so that your calves are on the seat of the chair. Your back, arms, and the backs of your hands should be on the floor. Raise your legs to vertical. If you stretch your arms over your head at this point, with your palms up, and pull your abdomen in, you are doing Urdva Prasarita Padasana (Upright Extended Foot Pose, known for reducing abdominal fat). This is also a modified version of Viparita Karani, the first pose in chapter 6, "Musculoskeletal Pain." In either pose, or in all, breathe easily for ten to fifteen seconds.

To exit, bend your knees so your shins are once again on the seat of the chair. Bring your left leg off the chair seat. Inch your way to a diagonal position with your left foot so that you can bring your right leg to the floor on the same side of the chair.

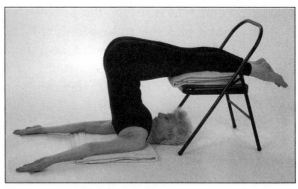

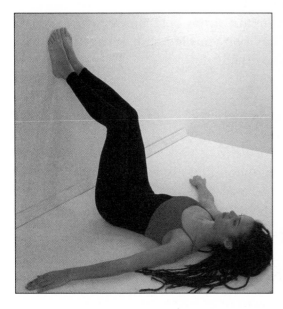

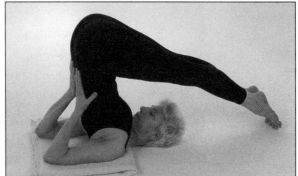

HALASANA MODIFIED (VERSION 2) Lie on the floor with a blanket or blankets under your shoulders (not your head). A chair should be placed a foot behind your head. Your hands are placed at your sides. As you bring your knees up to your chest, press your palms down on the floor and straighten your legs slightly to bring your thighs over your face and your shins onto the seat of the chair. Straighten your elbows, keeping them on the floor. Support your back with your palms. Bring your elbows in and press your hands against your back near your kidneys in order to keep your back more elevated. Arch your entire back slightly and raise your sit bones as high as possible.

Breathe with your mouth closed for ten to fifteen seconds. Keep your neck relaxed. While your shins are on the chair seat, gradually straighten your knees. As you get more proficient at this pose, you will be able to straighten them with less and less shin support.

To exit the pose, disengage your hands, but keep your arms extended behind you, hands far enough apart for your back to descend between them. Gradually bring your torso back to the floor, using arm pressure and abdominal strength to restrain and control the process. Keep your legs on the chair until you are quite a ways down. Then lift your feet only as far as necessary, continuing your descent until the sacrum is firmly on the floor. Only then should you lower your legs to the floor. You might want a helper the first few times you do this.

HALASANA REGULAR Do not use a chair. Lie on your back, arms at your sides, palms down beside your hips. Bend your knees as you raise your thighs to vertical. Then straighten the knees and push down on the floor with your palms to push your hips up as you lower your feet over your head. Keep pushing as the sacrum and lower back leave the floor and begin to rise. The weight of your feet will cantilever your pelvis higher and higher. The balance changes when your extended legs pass the horizontal and the feet descend as the pelvis rises. Continue until the toes touch the floor beyond your head.

Place the heels of your hands at the kidney region of the lower back, fingers pointed upward, elbows as close together as possible. Remember to arch your back slightly and raise the sit bones. Start at ten to fifteen seconds in this position, breathing as deeply as possible. Eventually you can stay in this pose for several minutes. One way to improve your inverted posture is to interlock your fingers and straighten out your elbows, pressing your entire arms against the floor. This rolls you onto the apex of your shoulders and further elevates the sit bones.

To exit, release your hands, bend your elbows, and replace your hands on your back in the vicinity of the kidneys. Let your torso descend into your hands, keeping your feet as close to the floor as possible. The feet will probably rise a little as your lower torso and pelvis come to the floor. Keep them low. Swing your legs up and over your head to vertical. Only after your back is securely on the floor should you bend your knees after your thighs come to vertical, then lower your thighs. Support yourself with your arms and hands while bringing your legs and feet down, but keep your neck fully relaxed.

Your head shouldn't leave the floor until you have finished the pose.

There are some poses that are described and pictured elsewhere in the book for other diagnoses that may also be helpful for weight control. These poses are listed in order of acute to chronic pain:

TRIKONASANA—Triangle Pose

TRIANGA MUKHAIKAPADA PASCHIMOTTANASANA—Three Limb Stretch to the West

MARICHYASANA I—Son of Brahma, Creator of the Universe

JATHARA PARIVARTANASANA—Rolling Stomach

CHAPTER 14

After Back Surgery

Just making the decision to have surgery is stressful. After the surgery itself, you wake up, usually in less pain than you were in before the procedure. Yet your body is responding in many ways to the invasion—yes, the violence—it has suffered. Your endocrine system usually takes a few days to get back to normal after surgery, peaking in its abnormal functions about one to two days after an operation. Literature suggests, and I have found, that yoga is a wonderful way to help yourself return to peak objective and subjective performance.[1]

Ideally you should begin a daily program of yoga practice before you undergo surgery. This will, of course, help increase your strength, your flexibility, and your stamina to undergo the procedure. If you haven't begun a yoga program before the operation, however, doing the asanas in the order in which they appear in this chapter will help you regain your strength after the operation. They will also aid in combating the emotional distress and depression that comes before surgery and may linger afterwards. If you are experiencing anxiety, either before or after a surgical procedure, meditation may be of use to you.

Following surgery, motion is most problematical near the site of the incision. Those muscles need the flexibility and strength that come from exercise. But strenuous exercise is usually forbidden after surgery to avoid possible reinjury.[2] I believe yoga is ideal because it can rely on isometric exercise. The principle of isometrics is that muscles contract and may be used in groups to increase strength, but there is no movement of joints, nor is there any impact. Because of this, yoga is unlikely to disrupt sutures, reactivate old injuries, or cause new ones.

In twenty years of experience with patients I have found that yoga is helpful for regulating gastrointestinal activity, including appetite. This is the direct result of work on the abdomen and also feedback from that work to the central nervous system. Many patients have told me it has been effective in reducing bloating and constipation, and adjusting appetite after surgery. Though I have never needed back surgery myself, I have had shoulder and abdominal procedures. I have found yoga has hastened my own recovery after anesthesia.

After surgery, although the original pain may have disappeared, the incisions can produce quite a bit of discomfort. Yoga teaches patients calm and control in the face of pain, one of the biggest problems after an operation. I have found that it may replace or augment medication in controlling pain, giving the patient a practical means of self-help.

How the Following Poses May Help

I suggest beginning with the first pose, Dandasana, and going on in order from there once you have had surgery. Most spinal procedures are done through the back. If you have had an abdominal incision, you must take more precautions and do any exercise, including yoga, with extra care. Check with your doctor before doing any exercise. Remember, a stretch may help you but not at the site of the incision.

- Begin slowly.
- Do poses once a day until balance and stamina begin to return.
- When possible, increase the length of time you hold a pose.
- When possible, do a pose up to three times daily.
- Wait four to five hours after eating to do the poses.

The reason an empty stomach is so important is that increased abdominal pressure and tilting and compressing maneuvers are so frequent in yoga poses. The stomach can become twisted and/or compressed. If that were to happen, its contents could be displaced in an upward or downward direction, weakening sphincters and causing further problems. I have found that if patients do poses on an empty stomach, that can aid in returning proper digestive functions and a healthy appetite.

Associated with any surgery is a certain amount of time you must spend resting in bed. One loses 20 percent of one's strength for each week in bed.[3] Exercise has been found to increase strength only 10 percent per week at most.[4] This means that every week of inactivity really represents three weeks of reduced strength. Yoga is a sensible and realistic method to help yourself return to normal functioning sooner, without elaborate equipment, without risk or cost, quietly, and at home.

1 . DANDASANA
Staff

BENEFITS: Safely strengthens lumbar and thoracic (lower and middle back) muscles and hip flexor muscles. Improves posture.

WARNING: If you have a spinal cord injury, MS, or ALS, use a wall. Otherwise this is a very safe pose.

DANDASANA Sit with legs parallel and in front of you, so you can feel the sit (ischial) bones. Knees are straight, ankles together, feet firmly vertical. Palms are on the floor close to hips. Back is erect. The erect back is the most important element of this pose. Breathe evenly, quietly, and symmetrically for ten to fifteen seconds.

To come out of this pose, relax your back and bend your knees.

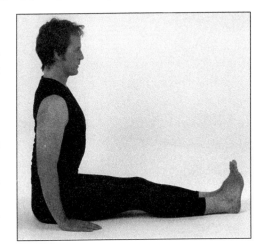

2. NAVASANA
Boat

BENEFITS: Strengthens and coordinates lumbar and abdominal and thigh muscles. Improves balance.

WARNING: Don't do this pose if you have an abdominal incision.

NAVASANA MODIFIED Begin the pose in Dandasana (1, above). Keeping your back straight, place your palms on the floor behind you, fingers pointing forward. Bend your left knee thirty degrees. Raise your left leg up off the floor several inches. At first it is easier to lift

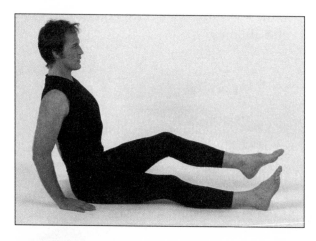

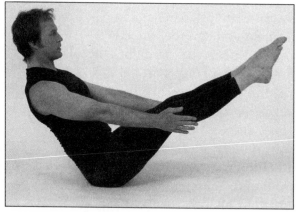

the bent knee higher. Hold the left leg up for ten to fifteen seconds, breathing evenly. Gradually, with repetitions and over time, straighten the knee while the leg is aloft. After breathing quietly for ten to fifteen seconds in the pose, gradually lower your leg until your foot is on the floor. Do this pose on both sides.

NAVASANA REGULAR Begin in Dandasana (1, above). Keeping back and legs straight, extend your arms horizontally in front of you, palms facing each other. Lift your legs thirty degrees as your straight torso reclines thirty degrees. Your legs still form a right angle with the torso. Shoulders are back and arms are extended in front of you, palms parallel to each other, arms horizontal. Your gaze will be perpendicular to your raised torso. Breathe in the whole chest, not just the top, for ten to fifteen seconds. Gradually increase the time you hold this pose to half a minute or a full minute.

To get out of this pose, relax your hands and place them at your sides and on the floor. Use them for support as you relax and slowly lower your legs.

3. APPROACH TO PADMASANA
Lotus

BENEFITS: Calming and relaxing. Helps with posture and is possible to do after back surgery. Stretches iliotibial bands, the muscles in the sides of the thighs.

WARNING: Beginners should do this, which is a way to get ready to do the Lotus pose, sitting in a Lotus position with one leg at a time. Begin with a painless position and gradually increase the stretch. Use caution if you have knee problems.

NOTE: It may seem strange to ask someone recently out of surgery to jump right into Lotus, a difficult pose and one advanced yogis hold in high esteem. Actually it is a safe, stable, and supremely calming pose, which explains both its suitability for doing after surgery and why yogis enjoy remaining in it for hours. The best advice for doing this and all the other postsurgery poses is: Think sharply, analyze intensely, but don't try too hard.

PADMASANA MODIFIED (VERSION 1) "Training for Lotus." Sit on the floor with your legs comfortably bent in front of you. Cradle your right foot in your hands; place it on the left thigh as high up toward the groin as you can. Bend the left leg and place it in front of you with the sole of the foot facing to the right and the knee bent so that your two shins are parallel. Your palms should be on the floor in front of you. Keep your back straight and head erect. Gently and slowly lean forward and slide your hands forward as you do, evenly distributing your weight on your knees. Stay there. Do not rock back and forth. Breathe smoothly, not jerkily, as you do this. Hold for twenty seconds.

To come out of this pose, bend forward slightly. Remove your right foot from your left groin. Reverse legs and do the pose on the other side.

PADMASANA MODIFIED (VERSION 2) Lying on your back with knees slightly bent, bring the right foot up to your hands by further bending the knee. Hold the foot firmly in both hands and place it as high up on the left thigh, as near to the left groin as possible. Now

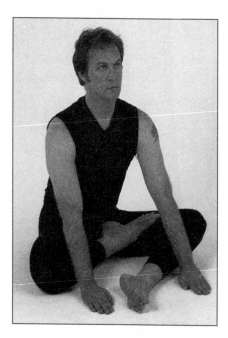

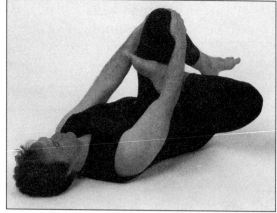

flex the left hip and bend the left knee sufficiently to bring either the thigh or the shin within your reach. Grasp the thigh or shin or knee with both hands and steadily pull it toward your chin. If you have had left-knee difficulties, grasp the thigh, not the knee or shin. Do not raise your head; lie with back, ribs, and head relaxed and flat on the floor. When you have reached an amount of pull and stretch that begins to be painful or exhausting, hold it there for ten to fifteen seconds, bringing your shoulders back, together, and down toward your waist. Breathe slowly.

To leave the pose, let your left thigh come down by first extending your elbows. Then release the left leg, remove the right foot from the left groin, and repeat on the other side.

4. TADASANA
Mountain

BENEFITS: Calming. Helpful for balance and posture.

WARNING: If dizziness occurs, do the pose standing close to a wall.

NOTE: To remain motionless requires concentration and determination every time you attempt it.

TADASANA MODIFIED Stand with your feet parallel to each other, in a line with your hips and shoulders. Balance your weight between the feet and within each foot. Do not arch your back or hunch your shoulders. Straighten your knees. Spread your toes out like a fan. Balance weight evenly between your feet—the front and back, inside and outside of each foot. Stand totally still. Breathe quietly for thirty seconds.

Believe it or not, it is difficult to come out of this pose. It's not clear exactly what you have to do to stop standing still, except that you begin to move. I believe it is important to recognize the calm, relaxation, and peace you are leaving behind.

TADASANA REGULAR Standing in the modified pose, interlock your fingers. Extend your hands and arms over your head, especially elevating the pulpy part of the hands near the thumbs. Stretch

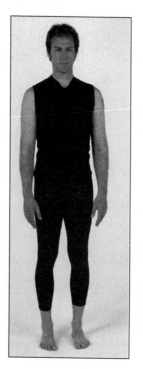
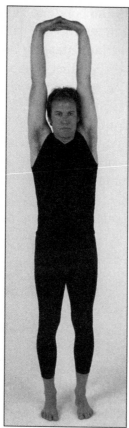

the entire back of the body. Bring your arms up above your head. Stretch upward, with palms facing the ceiling. Stand motionless for up to thirty seconds.

To leave this pose, gradually and symmetrically bring your hands to your sides, without losing your balance. Stand motionless for a few moments.

5. BADDHA KONASANA I
Bound Angle

BENEFITS: Improves pelvic circulation. Relieves sciatica. Good for menstrual cramps, bloating, and menstrual regularity.

WARNING: After your surgery, or if you have hip arthritis, begin doing this pose gradually. Avoid doing this pose if you have had abdominal incisions or sacroiliac derangement.

BADDHA KONASANA I MODIFIED Sit on the floor with knees bent, soles touching and heels as close as possible. Interlock your fingers. Hold your feet. Keep your back straight. Lean forward, pressing your elbows into the crevices between calves and thighs on both sides. Go as far as is comfortable. Press your legs outward and down. Breathe slowly and deeply for ten to fifteen seconds.

To leave this pose, walk with your fingertips toward your torso. Keeping your back straight, come to the upright position. Place your hands outside your thighs in line with your buttocks. Straighten both knees.

BADDHA KONASANA I REGULAR Sit on the floor with the knees bent and the outsides of the thighs as close to the floor as possible. Soles of the feet are touching; heels are close together between your thighs. Interlock your fingers around the little-toe sides of the joined feet. Bring your shoulders back, elbows close to your sides. Keeping your back straight, lower your solar plexis to the soles of your feet.

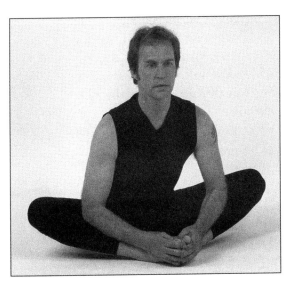 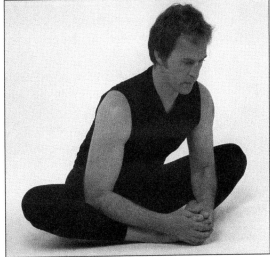

Rest your forehead on the floor, only if you've come forward enough to do so without bending your neck or hunching forward. In any case, your head may tilt back but your neck should remain straight. Breathe quietly for ten to fifteen seconds after coming forward as much as possible.

To exit this pose, gradually release the pressure of your hands on the outsides of your feet. Keeping your head up and your back straight, gradually come to the seated position. Release feet.

6. VIRABHADRASANA II
Warrior Pose II

BENEFITS: Strengthens entire back, neck, and shoulders. Strengthens legs.

WARNING: If necessary for balance, do this pose against a wall. Do not do this pose if you are pregnant.

VIRABHADRASANA II MODIFIED Stand with feet four to five feet apart. The taller you are, the farther apart your feet should be. As you inhale, raise your arms to horizontal, palms down, hands concave upwards. Turn your left foot out ninety degrees. Turn your right foot in thirty degrees. Your navel should face straight ahead. Keeping your right knee straight, bend your left knee as far as is comfortable. Keep the torso upright as you descend. Don't hang back or lunge forward. Stay vertical, hands even. Distribute your weight equally between your two legs. Turn your head to the left, without bending it forward or tilting it. Sight along your left thumb. Stay in the pose for ten to fifteen seconds, breathing evenly.

To exit this pose straighten your left knee, then turn your feet straight ahead and parallel. As you exhale bring your arms to your sides, or go directly into the pose on the other side.

VIRABHADRASANA II REGULAR Bend left knee ninety degrees so your shin is vertical and your left thigh is horizontal. Stretch your fingertips as far apart as possible and widen your chest.

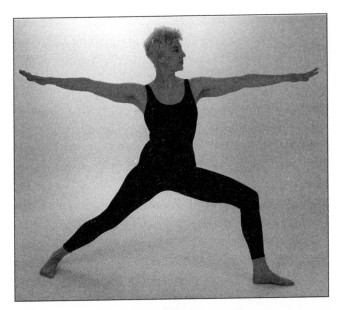

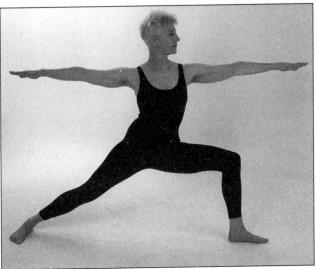

Keeping your torso and arms in one straight vertical plane, gradually straighten your left knee to come out of this pose. Bring your arms down, feet forward. As you exhale, gradually release your hands. Repeat on the other side.

There are some poses that are described and pictured elsewhere in the book for other diagnoses that may also be helpful after surgery. These poses are listed in order of acute to chronic pain:

VIRASANA—Hero Pose

SUPTA PADANAGUSTHASANA—Holding Big Toe While Supine

ANANTASANA—Vishnu's Couch

UTKATASANA—Intense Forward Bend

NOTES

CHAPTER 1

1. L. G. Hart, R. A. Deyo, and D. C. Cherkin, "Physician Office Visits for Low Back Pain: Frequency, Clinical Evaluation, and Treatment Patterns from a U.S. National Survey," *Spine* 20, no. 1 (January 1995): 11–19.

2. G. B. J. Andersson, "The Epidemiology of Spinal Disorders," in *The Adult Spine: Principles and Practice*, ed. J. W. Frymoyer (New York: Raven Press, 1991) 107–46. R. A. Sternback, "Survey of Pain in the United States: The Nuprin Report," *Clinical Journal of Pain* 2, no. 4 (1986): 49–53.

3. L. DiPietro, T. E. Seeman, N. S. Stachenfelt, et al., "Moderate-Intensity Aerobic Training Improves Glucose Responses in Aging Independent of Abdominal Adiposity," *Journal of the American Geriatrics Society* 46 (July 1998): 875–79.

4. O. Yanagisawa, M. Niitsu, et al., "MRI Determination of Muscle Recruitment Variations in Dynamic Ankle Plantar Flexion Exercise," *American Journal of Physical Medicine and Rehabilitation* 82, no. 10 (October 2003): 760–65.

5. M. S. Garfinkel, H. R. Schumacher Jr., et al., "Evaluation of a Yoga-Based Regimen for Treatment of Osteoarthritis of the Hands," *Journal of Rheumatology* 21, no. 12 (December 1994): 2341–43.

6. M. Dash and S. Telles, "Improvement in Hand-Grip Strength in Normal Volunteers and Rheumatoid Arthritis Patients Following Yoga Training," *Indian Journal of Physiological Pharmacology* 45, no. 3 (July 2001): 355–60. J. E. Stevens, R. L. Mizner, and L. Snyder-Mackler, "Quadriceps Strength and Volitional Activation before and after Total Knee Arthroplasty for Osteoarthritis," *Journal of Orthopedic Research* 21, no. 5 (September 2003): 775–79.

7. Comment on L. A. Danneels, G. G. Vanderstraeten, D. C. Cambier, et al., "Effects of Three Different Training Modalities on the Cross Sectional Area of the Lumbar Multifidus Muscle in Patients with Chronic Low Back Pain," *British Journal of Sports Medicine* 37, no. 1 (February 2003): 91.

8. H. Sekiguchi, K. Nakazawa, and S. Suzuki, "Differences in Recruitment Properties of the Corticospinal Pathway between Lengthening and Shortening Contractions in Human Soleus Muscle," *Brain Research* 977, no. 2 (July 2003): 169–79.

9. S. C. Lanyon, *Osteoporosis and Exercise: Topics in Geriatric Rehabilitation,* March 1989, Aspen Press, 4 (2): 12–24.

10. Herbert Benson with Miriam Z. Klipper, *The Relaxation Response* (New York: Morrow, 1974).

11. B.K.S. Iyengar, *Light on Pranayama: The Yogic Art of Breathing* (New York: Crossroad, 1995). Mira Mehta, *How to Use Yoga: A Step-by-Step Guide to the Iyengar Method of Yoga, for Relaxation, Health and Well-Being* (Berkeley, Calif.: Rodmell Press, 1998).

12. B. Balasubramanian and M. S. Pansare, "Effect of Yoga on Aerobic and Anaerobic Power of Muscles," *Indian Journal of Physiological Pharmacology* 35, no. 4 (October 1991): 281–82. O. P. Bhatnagar and V. Anantharaman, "The Effect of Yoga Training on Neuromuscular Excitability and Muscular Relaxation," *Neurology India* 25, no. 4 (December 1977): 230–32. P. Raghuraj and S. Telles, "Muscle Power, Dexterity Skill and Visual Perception in Community Home Girls Trained in Yoga or Sports and in Regular School Girls," *Indian Jour-*

nal of Physiology and Pharmacology 41, no. 4 (October 1997): 409–15. R. Vyas and N. Dikshit, "Effect of Meditation on Respiratory System, Cardiovascular System and Lipid Profile," *Indian Journal of Physiology and Pharmacology* 46, no. 4 (October 2002): 487–91. A. Malathi, A. Damodaran, et al., "Effect of Yogic Practices on Subjective Well-Being," *Indian Journal of Physiology and Pharmacology* 44, no. 2 (April 2000): 202–6. R. La Forge, "Mind-Body Fitness: Encouraging Prospects for Primary and Secondary Prevention," *Journal of Cardiovascular Nursing* 11, no. 3 (April 1977): 53–65.

CHAPTER 2

1. Dean Ornish, *Dr. Dean Ornish's Program for Reversing Heart Disease: The Only System Scientifically Proven to Reverse Heart Disease Without Drugs or Surgery* (New York: Random House, 1996). Michael Lerner, *Choices in Healing: Integrating the Best of Conventional and Complementary Approaches to Cancer* (Cambridge, Mass.: MIT Press, 1994).

CHAPTER 3

1. Andrew Thomas, "Yoga and Fascia," *The Journal of the International Association of Yoga Therapists*, no. 3 (1992): 39–42.

CHAPTER 4

1. BBC News World Edition, "Yoga Injuries Increasing," 9 September 2002.

2. Linda Camras, Harriet Oster, et al., "Emotional Facial Expressions in European-American, Japanese, and Chinese Infants," *Annals of the New York Academy of Sciences* 1,000 (2003): 135–51.

3. John E. Sarno, *Healing Back Pain: The Mind-Body Connection* (New York: Warner Books, 1991).

4. K. G. Davis, W. S. Marras, et al., "The Impact of Mental Processing and Pacing on Spine Loading," *Spine* 27, no. 3 (December 2002): 2645–53.

5. Ernest Holmes, *The Science of Mind* (New York: R. M. McBride, 1938). Harold G. Koenig, *The Healing Power of Faith: Science Explores Medicine's Last Great Frontier* (New York: Simon & Schuster, 1999). Larry Dossey, *Prayer Is Good Medicine: How to Reap the Healing Benefits of Prayer* (San Francisco: HarperSanFrancisco, 1996).

CHAPTER 5

1. National Institutes of Health BMI (body mass index) available at http://nhlbisupport.com/bmi/bmicalc.htm (accessed 1 March 2004).

2. Rene Cailliet, *Soft Tissue Pain and Disability*, 2d ed. (Philadelphia: F. A. Davis Company, 1988).

3. R. A. Deyo, J. Rainville, and D. L. Kent, "What Can the History and Physical Examination Tell Us about Low Back Pain?" *Journal of the American Medical Association* 268, no. 6 (August 1992): 760–65.

4. Garfinkel and Schumacher, "Evaluation of a Yoga-Based Regimen." M. Garfinkel and H. R. Schumacher, Jr., "Yoga," *Rheumatic Diseases Clinics of North America* 26, no. 1 (February 2000): 125–32.

CHAPTER 7

1. Maureen C. Jensen, Michael N. Brant-Zawadzki, et al., "Magnetic Resonance Imaging of the Lumbar Spine in People without Back Pain," *New England Journal of Medicine* 331, no. 2 (July 1994): 69–73.

CHAPTER 8

1. For more information, see the Arthritis Foundation Web site at www.arthritis.org/conditions/diseasecenter (accessed 1 March 2004).

2. Ibid.

3. M. Garfinkel and H. R. Schumacher, Jr., "Yoga." *Rheumatic Diseases Clinics of North America*, February 2000, 26 (1): 125–32.

4. J. Kabat-Zinn, "An Outpatient Program in Behavioral Medicine for Chronic Pain Patients Based on the Practice of Mindfulness Meditation: Theoretical Considerations and Preliminary Results," *General Hospital Psychiatry* 4, no. 1 (April 1982): 33–47.

CHAPTER 9

1. Avital Fast, "Low Back Pain During Pregnancy," in *Low Back Pain Handbook: A Practical Guide for the Primary Care Physician*, eds. Andrew J. Cole and Stanley A. Herring (Philadelphia: Hanley and Belfus, 1997), 345–51.

CHAPTER 10

1. M. J. Mantle, R. M. Greenwood, and H. L. Currey, "Backache in Pregnancy," *Rheumatology and Rehabilitation* 16, no. 2 (1977): 95–101.

2. Sally Kempton, *The Heart of Meditation: Pathways to a Deeper Experience* (South Fallsburg, N.Y.: SYDA Foundation, 2002).

CHAPTER 11

1. H. Koike, "The Extensibility of Aplysia Nerve and the Determination of True Axon Length," *Journal of Physiology* 390, no. 1 (September 1987): 469–87. S. Tani, S. Yamada, and R. S. Knighton, "Extensibility of the Lumbar and Sacral Cord: Pathophysiology of the Tethered Spinal Cord in Cats," *Journal of Neurosurgery* 66, no. 1 (January 1987): 116–23.

CHAPTER 12

1. Jane Brody, "Personal Health, A Sciatic Villain that Eludes Detection," *New York Times*, 15 April 1992, Section C, 14.

2. L. M. Fishman, G. W. Dombi, et al., "Piriformis Syndrome: Diagnosis, Treatment, and Outcome—A 10-Year Study," *Archives of Physical Medicine and Rehabilitation* 83, no. 3 (March 2002): 295–301. L. M. Fishman, C. Anderson, and B. Rosner, "Botox and Physical Therapy in the Treatment of Piriformis Syndrome," *American Journal of Physical Medicine and Rehabilitation* 81, no. 12 (December 2000): 936–42.

3. L. M. Fishman, L. M. Konnoth, et al., "Botulinim neurotoxin type B and physical therapy in the treatment of piriformis syndrome: a dose-finding study," *American Journal of Physical Medicine and Rehabilitation* 83, no. 1 (January 2004): 42–50.

CHAPTER 13

1. M. D. Tran, R. G. Holly, et al., "Effects of Hatha Yoga Practice on the Health-Related Aspects of Physical Fitness," *Preventive Cardiolology* 4, no. 4 (Autumn 2001): 165–70.

CHAPTER 14

1. Balasubramanian and Pansare, "Effect of Yoga." H. H. Handoll, M. J. Parker, and C. Sherrington, "Mobilisation Strategies after Hip Fracture Surgery in Adults," *Cochrane Database System Review* 2003, issue 1: CD001704.

2. G. Spahn, R. Wittig, ["Biomechanical Properties (compressive strength and pressure at break) of hyaline cartilage under axial load"], *Zentralblatt fur Chirurgie* (January 2003): 78–82.

3. J. E. Stevens, et al., "Quadriceps strength and volitional activation before and after total knee arthroplasty for osteoarthritis," *Journal of Orthopaedic Research* 21, no. 5 (September 2003): 775–79.

4. U. S. Ray, B. Sinha, et al., "Aerobic Capacity and Perceived Exertion after Practice of Hatha Yogic Exercises," *Indian Journal of Medical Research* 114 (December 2001): 215–21.

SUGGESTED READING

Cole, Andrew J., and Stanley A. Herring, eds. *Low Back Pain Handbook: A Practical Guide for the Primary Care Physician.* Philadelphia: Hanley and Belfus, 1997.

Dillard, James N., with Leigh Ann Hirschman. *The Chronic Pain Solution: The Comprehensive, Step-by-Step Guide to Choosing the Best of Alternative and Conventional Medicine.* New York: Bantam Books, 2002.

Dossey, Larry. *Prayer Is Good Medicine: How to Reap the Healing Benefits of Prayer.* San Francisco: HarperSanFrancisco, 1996.

Dunkin, Mary Anne. *All You Need to Know about Back Pain: Increase Your Mobility, Know Your Options.* Atlanta: Arthritis Foundation, 2002.

Fishman, Loren, and Carol Ardman. *Back Pain: How to Relieve Low Back Pain and Sciatica.* New York: W. W. Norton and Company, 1999.

Hatha Yoga Pradipika. [Many translations available.]

Holmes, Ernest. *The Science of Mind.* New York: R. M. McBride, 1938.

Iyengar, B.K.S. *Light on Yoga: Yoga Dipika.* New York: Schocken Books, 1966.

Jordan, Sandra. *Yoga for Pregnancy: Safe and Gentle Stretches.* New York: St. Martin's Press, 1987.

Kempton, Sally. *The Heart of Meditation: Pathways to a Deeper Experience.* South Fallsburg, N.Y.: SYDA Foundation, 2002.

Lasater, Judith. *Relax and Renew: Restful Yoga for Stressful Times.* Berkeley, Calif.: Rodmell Press, 1995.

Payne, Larry, and Richard Usatine. *Yoga Rx: A Step-by-Step Program to Promote Health, Wellness, and Healing for Common Ailments.* New York: Broadway Books, 2002.

Sarno, John E. *Healing Back Pain: The Mind-Body Connection.* New York: Warner Books, 1991.

Schatz, Mary Pullig. *Back Care Basics: A Doctor's Gentle Yoga Program for Back and Neck Pain Relief.* Berkeley, Calif.: Rodmell Press, 1992.

Sparrowe, Linda, and Patricia Walden. *The Woman's Book of Yoga and Health: A Lifelong Guide to Wellness.* Boston: Shambhala, 2002.

Taimni, I. K. *The Science of Yoga: A Commentary on the Yoga-Sutras of Patanjali in the Light of Modern Thought.* Wheaton, Ill.: Theosophical Publishing House, 1967.

Weller, Stella. *The Yoga Back Book: The Gentle Yet Effective Way to Spinal Health.* Rev. ed. London: Thorsons, 2000.

White, Augustus A. *Your Aching Back: A Doctor's Guide to Relief.* New York: Simon & Schuster, 1990.

White, Augustus A., and Manohar M. Panjabi. *Clinical Biomechanics of the Spine.* 2d ed. Philadelphia: Lippincott, 1990.

RESOURCES

Yoga Teachers and Yoga Therapists

The International Association of Yoga Therapists
109 Hillside
Mill Valley, CA 94941
(415) 383-4587
www.YREC.org

Ashtanga Yoga
The Yoga Workshop
2020 21st Street
Boulder, CO 80302
(303) 449-6102
www.yogaworkshop.com

American Viniyoga Institute
PO Box 88
Makawao, HI 96768
Phone: (808) 572-1414
Fax: (808) 573-2000
www.Viniyoga.com

Anusara Yoga
9400 Grogans Mill Rd., Ste. 200
The Woodlands, TX 77380
Toll free: 1-888-398-9642
Local: (281) 367-9763
oneyoga@anusara.com

Svaroopa Yoga
Master Yoga Foundation
450 Pearl Street
La Jolla, CA 92017
info@masteryoga.org
e-mail: *info@masteryoga.org*

The Phoenix Rising Center
West Stockbridge, MA 01266
1-800-288-9642
www.pryc.com

British Wheel of Yoga
25 Jermyn Street
Sleaford
Lincolnshire, England NG34 7RU
Tel: 01529 306 851
Fax: 01529 303 233
email: *office@bwy.org.uk*

Yoga Equipment

Yoga.com
(866) 266-YOGA
information, videos, books, equipment, clothing
www.gaiam.com
videos, books, equipment, clothing

Author's Web Site on Back Pain

www.Sciatica.org
back pain information from Loren Fishman, MD

ABOUT THE AUTHORS

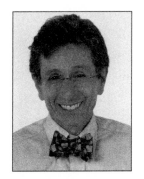

LOREN FISHMAN, MD, is a graduate of Christ Church, Oxford, where he studied philosophy. He graduated from Rush Medical School, trained at Harvard-Tufts, and did his residency at Albert Einstein College of Medicine. He studied yoga with B.K.S. Iyengar and has been practicing yoga for thirty years; he regularly uses yoga in his medical practice. Dr. Fishman has authored and published more than fifty academic papers in the philosophy of science and in his specialty, rehabilitation medicine. He is associate editor of *Topics in Geriatric Rehabilitation* and the coauthor of a previous book, *Low Back Pain: How to Relieve Low Back Pain and Sciatica*. In addition, he is on the staff at Columbia-Presbyterian Hospital in New York City and is in private practice. A frequent lecturer and interview subject, Dr. Fishman has also appeared on national television as a back pain expert.

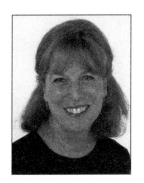

CAROL ARDMAN is a writer and editor specializing in health and medicine. She is coauthor, with Dr. Fishman, of *Low Back Pain: How to Relieve Low Back Pain and Sciatica*. Her many articles have appeared in the *New York Times*, *Ms.* magazine, *Boston* magazine, the *New York Daily News*, and numerous holistic health magazines, professional journals, and Web sites. As an editorial and media consultant, she has been instrumental in launching new publications in the complementary and alternative medicine field.

ABOUT THE MODELS

SALLY HESS was born and raised in New York City and began her dance career as the Child in Doris Humphrey's *Day on Earth with José Limon*. She has danced at home and abroad with many moderndance companies and performs her solo works worldwide. Sally studied with Joan White and became a Certified Yoga Instructor (1996) in the method of B.K.S. Iyengar. She is an associate professor in the Department of Music and Dance at Swarthmore College.

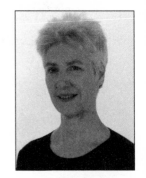

JENNIFER HICKS earned a B.S. in physical therapy from the University of South Alabama in 1999, fulfilling her lifetime goal. She is now practicing in a private rehabilitation practice in New York City. Neurological rehabilitation and manual therapy are Jennifer's special interests. In the future she would like to become certified in manual therapy. Jennifer has only recently begun to practice yoga, but she is enthusiastic about pursuing yoga, both for herself and her patients. A native of Madison, Alabama, Jennifer lives in Brooklyn, New York.

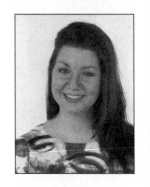

NICKI MARSHALL is a Vermont native who graduated with a B.A. in dance from Mount Holyoke College in 2000. She was certified as a hatha vinyasa yoga instructor in the fall of 2002, and teaches yoga in New York City. A modern and African dancer and choreographer, Nicki teaches dance through the National Dance Institutes and the Brooklyn Arts Exchange.

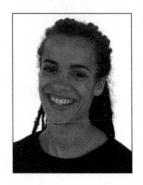

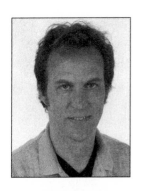

MICHAEL NOLAN is a registered movement therapist and educator with a background in modern dance. He has been involved in movement arts as a trainer, teacher, performer, and student for more than twenty years. Michael describes his work in yoga as "an ongoing process of self-discovery and professional development." He lives in Brooklyn, New York, with his son, Graham.

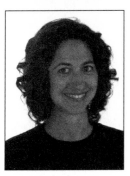

MIRIAM ADLER BRAM is a certified holistic nutritional counselor and the founder of Eating for Two (*www.eatfortwo.com*), which provides personalized nutritional programs for pregnant women with the goal of creating positive choices in diet and lifestyle to support a healthy pregnancy. She trained at the Institute for Integrative Nutrition in New York and received her B.A. in psychology from the University of Michigan. An avid yogi, Miriam lives in Katonah, New York, with her husband and daughter, Zoe.